THE COMPLETE BOOK OF LASER EYE SURGERY

Stephen G. Slade, M.D.
with Richard N. Baker, O.D.
and Dorothy Kay Brockman

Foreword by
Spencer P. Thornton, M.D.
former President, American Society
of Cataract and Refractive Surgery

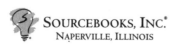

SOURCEBOOKS, INC.
NAPERVILLE, ILLINOIS

Published by Sourcebooks, Inc.
P.O. Box 4410, Naperville, Illinois 60567-4410
(630) 961-3900
FAX: 630-961-2168

Library of Congress Cataloging-in-Publication Data

Slade, Stephen, 1953-
    The complete book of laser eye surgery / Stephen G. Slade, Richard N.
    Baker, Dorothy Kay Brockman.
      p. cm.
    Includes index.
    ISBN 1-57071-633-1 (alk. paper)
      1. LASIK (Eye surgery) 2. Eye—Laser surgery. I Baker, Richard N. II.
      Brockman, Dorothy. III. Title

RE336.S93 2000
617.7"55—dc21
                                                                00-044043

Printed and bound in the United States of America

·VHG   10 9 8 7 6 5 4 3 2 1

This book is dedicated to three women of
great courage—our mothers.

Nell Rowan Slade
Mable Baker
Violet Rose Hammers

Having LASIK is a journey from a dreary, dimly lit room filled with formless shadows into the bright, glorious sunlight on the most beautiful day of your life.

CONTENTS

LIST OF
ILLUSTRATIONS

FOREWORD

For millions of nearsighted persons and those with other refractive errors, vision correction surgery offers a way to eliminate or reduce dependence on glasses and contact lenses. Today, several million people around the world can see better as a result of the astonishing advances in computerized excimer laser technology. Over the past twenty years, many people have improved their vision with the older, non-laser-based procedure called radial keratotomy, or RK. In the near future, laser refractive surgeries, which are more accurate, may become the most popular of all ophthalmic procedures.

Before having any refractive operation, patients need expert answers concerning all the potential benefits and risks of these ever-evolving surgical techniques. Today, people want to know precisely what happens when a surgeon permanently refocuses their eyes. No longer do patients merely ask their ophthalmologist, "Can you help me see better?" They want the tools to be able to participate in their health-care decisions. They want to know how their eyes work. They want to understand their diagnosis. They want to know exactly how excimer laser surgery can improve their vision and why it might work better than RK. And, most important of all, they want detailed answers about their individual chances for better eyesight.

To find answers to these questions, patients need a physician who is experienced in vision correction surgery—a doctor who follows the latest developments in this complex, technology-based field. If you are considering eye surgery, the relationship between you and your doctor is a special one. Your eyes are as unique as your fingerprints. Your surgeon and your individual healing response will determine your vision for the rest of your life. Your doctor must help you understand the surgery that is designed to allow you to overcome poor vision. Not only should you have a thorough eye examination with the latest ophthalmic instruments, but you also deserve your physician's complete attention during his time with you. You must make absolutely certain that he clearly understands your visual goals and needs.

Though your eye doctor and his staff may be totally committed to answering your questions, the spontaneous spoken word is seldom as well thought out and detailed as the written word. Hence, even if your physician spent hours explaining refractive eye surgery to you, he probably would be unable to present a totally clear and comprehensive picture of these procedures. For this reason, Dr. Stephen G. Slade, Dr. Richard N. Baker, and Dorothy Kay Brockman have designed this book to help you make informed decisions concerning your eyes. They want you to have an absolutely realistic grasp of what can and cannot be done to try to improve your vision. Offering clear explanations in easy-to-read language, the authors "sit down" with you and present an in-depth look at all the latest life-changing breakthroughs in this highly specialized field.

This book answers your questions about the newest laser eye surgery, known as LASIK, and about all of the other types of refractive eye surgery, including the original laser-based PRK (photorefractive keratectomy) procedure and the older RK (radial keratotomy) operation. An entire chapter is devoted to comparing the merits of these *procedures. The authors also discuss the chances of attaining better vision during an enhancement procedure to fine-tune the first refractive operation.*

Having performed thousands of laser vision correction operations, Dr. Slade—who helped perfect the modern LASIK microsurgical procedure—is uniquely qualified to write this book. The first to perform this state-of-the-art surgery as it is practiced worldwide today, he has taught refractive surgical techniques to thousands of eye doctors. Dedicated to preventing the misuse of refractive technology, he travels around the world teaching LASIK to ophthalmologists.

Dr. Baker has devoted most of his long professional career to helping Dr. Slade care for patients. This optometrist's experience in meeting the needs of tens of thousands of pre- and post-operative refractive surgery patients has given him great insight into the special concerns of people undergoing eye operations. Both doctors understand that fine eye care involves far more than reshaping the window of each eye with a laser.

Far from an impersonal medical text, The Complete Book of Laser Eye Surgery *is about people who have undergone an operation to improve their vision. By following other patients' struggles to overcome nearsightedness, farsightedness, or astigmatism, you will be better equipped to face the anxiety that usually accompanies any operation, but especially eye surgery. Even though the printed word can never replace the individualized support of your personal doctor, with this book at your side, you will have a better chance of realizing your long-awaited dream—the dream of excellent vision without glasses or contact lenses.*

Spencer P. Thornton, M.D., FACS
Former President
American Society of Cataract and Refractive Surgery

Author's Note

We have written this book to help you understand some of the fundamental aspects about how the eye works and about how vision correction surgery can reduce refractive errors such as nearsightedness, farsightedness, and astigmatism. Our goal is to provide you with basic background information to enable you to work more effectively with your personal doctor. No book for a general audience can advise you about your individual case—only your eye doctor can do that. Although we discuss many of the benefits and risks of refractive surgery, only a detailed medical book for ophthalmologists and optometrists can begin to cover all the possible rare complications that might occur following eye surgery. No two patients are alike—nor do they respond to surgery in the same way. Hence, before following any procedure covered in these chapters, you must consult your own physician.

Some stories here are based on actual cases, although details have been changed to protect patient identity. To picture a procedure more realistically, some stories are based on a combination of many cases.

ACKNOWLEDGMENTS

For taking the time to review specific chapters of this book, we wish to thank:

Spencer P. Thornton, M.D., and Richard L. Lindstrom, M.D.

We also wish to express our appreciation to our research assistant, Sabra Hargrove, who helped prepare the outlines and the glossary of this book and to our executive assistant, Cathy Ross, who managed countless details.

For making our book come alive with pictures, we thank our superb medical illustrators, Linda Warren and Jan Redden.

For recognizing the need for a readable book on LASIK eye surgery, we thank our literary agent, Heide Lange, vice president of Sanford J. Greenburger Associates. We also are extremely grateful to professor Ted Stanton, University of Houston, who was one of our copy editors, to our book editor, Hillel Black, and our project editor, Alex Lubertozzi, at Sourcebooks, Inc.

Finally, we owe much thanks to all the members of Dr. Slade's and Dr. Baker's staff, especially their multilingual center director, Eleticia Szozda, Dr. Slade's "Boss."

AUTHOR TO READER

My co-authors and I have written this book to help you understand the amazing new eye surgeries that are designed to improve vision. We cover all the current "refractive surgeries" that refocus the eye to make people less dependent on glasses and contact lenses. You will follow an extremely nearsighted person named "Karen" as she has the popular microsurgical procedure called LASIK—the excimer laser operation offering excellent results for nearsightedness, farsightedness, and astigmatism. This surgery can help you see better by permanently changing the curvature and thus the focusing power of the cornea, the eye's thin, transparent "window" that covers the dark, round pupil and colored iris.

In the hands of an expert, LASIK is a nearly ideal procedure. A specially trained eye doctor, using an automated surgical instrument, cuts a thin flap of surface cornea sideways across the anesthetized eye and folds back the tissue, which remains attached at one edge like a page of a book. A computer-driven laser light scalpel sculpts the inner cornea, removing only a tiny amount of tissue. Controlled by highly refined software, the cool ultraviolet laser beam reshapes the clear corneal lens for better vision. Each pulse removes only one quarter of a micron (one millionth of a meter). The surgeon carefully replaces the protective flap so that the delicate corneal surface is preserved. Images now focus more clearly on the retina (the brain's light-sensing receptors inside the back of the eye). Causing minimal discomfort, this operation is easy on the patient. Eyesight improves quickly. Many patients return to work the next day.

Millions of people will have this procedure in the next few years, yet only a few understand these operations. Some people decide to have laser surgery after reading a short magazine article, after a couple clicks on the Internet, or after a twenty-minute consultation with an eye doctor. Few would buy a car based on such limited information, yet untold numbers of people put their eyes under the laser after hearing one friend's glowing recommendation. Some even "have their eyes done" on a lunch break at the nearest shopping mall.

Most LASIK patients will be happy with their results. Their first reaction often is, "Wow! I can see the numbers on the wall clock without glasses." But even though laser surgery seems like a miracle, any operation on the human body has risks. Before having LASIK, people should know how it works and how to choose a doctor. Yet some patients say, "Surgery scares me. Spare me the details. Just get on with it." Well, they are talking about their precious vision. I believe that if you are considering laser surgery, you should understand all the known risks as well as the wonderful benefits.

This book strives to present such detailed knowledge in clear language that is accessible to patients. You not only will learn about modern LASIK, but also about the new custom version based on "wavefront" technology that promises improved results. In addition, you will read about all the other refractive surgeries that refocus the eye such as PRK, or photorefractive keratectomy (the original, or surface laser, operation), and RK, or radial keratotomy (the older, non-laser incisional procedure in which the surgeon creates partial-thickness cuts in the cornea with a diamond-tipped knife). We carefully compare LASIK, PRK, and RK in chapter 10, "Choosing the Right Refractive Surgery for You: LASIK, PRK, or RK." Although it is slightly more technical than the rest of the book, this chapter presents an in-depth insight into refractive surgery formerly available only in medical books.

We have devoted several chapters to enhancement procedures—second surgeries designed to refine original results. Although an additional operation has helped many patients, the risks are significantly greater the second time around. Doctors are unable to promise perfect vision to their patients by performing more surgery.

You probably have heard about some of the newest, ever-changing peripheral technologies to correct vision. We examine the benefits and risks of these procedures, some of which are still in clinical trials—always considering patient comfort and recovery time. An operation known as "corneal ring implantation surgery" has received much news coverage. During this procedure to correct mild nearsightedness, the surgeon slips two plastic, crescent-shaped arcs inside the cornea's middle layer near its circular edge. Another operation that we describe in detail is cataract surgery, a non-laser operation to replace a clouded crystalline lens (it's behind the cornea) with a clear artificial one. It can change the eye's focusing power for older people.

Only a comprehensive book can begin to show realistically the promise of refractive surgery—the power of these highly-technical, life-changing procedures to correct focusing errors such as common nearsightedness. Unfortunately, many people are learning about the popular state-of-the-art LASIK operation through mass advertising campaigns. Some marketing methods can be misleading. Although "sound-bite" commercials help make people aware of this innovative technology, they are unable to tell the whole story. For example, TV and radio advertisements seldom explain refractive surgery's effect on age-related presbyopia (a condition causing blurry near vision that affects middle-aged and older people). Nor can short commercials present details about potential complications.

Many LASIK newspaper articles begin with a happy story about a thrilled patient praising their new miracle vision and end with a sad case about a different person with a poor result. While most people get excellent results, problems absolutely do occur. Complication rates can vary considerably among doctors, depending upon their surgical skill, their training, and their understanding of their laser. A corneal surgeon—an ophthalmologist specially trained to operate within the cornea's multiple layers—may have an advantage performing LASIK. The newer flying-spot lasers may decrease the chance of problems.

Statistics can be confusing. You may wonder what is covered in the "complication rate." Does it include "undercorrections" where the patient's eyesight after surgery remains a little near- or far-sighted? What is the rate of rare serious infections that must be treated immediately with antibiotics? Are the complications temporary or permanent? Can they be surgically corrected? As we cover in detail, some complications can be managed immediately during the surgery, some are temporary, and some can be permanent.

We want you to be able to select a doctor with the lowest possible complication rates for the procedure that you are considering. Keep in mind that a physician may have a distinguished career in general ophthalmology, yet still be inexperienced at performing LASIK. As we stress throughout this book, LASIK looks deceptively easy to perform, but it requires great technical finesse. The surgeon's learning-curve is steep and endless. In our opinion, LASIK has the potential to help millions of people, but as I tell ophthalmologists at refractive surgery courses, the reputation of a procedure is only as good as its worst results. As much as humanly possible, doctors and their informed patients must reduce surgical risks to a minimum.

You may be fascinated with the idea of improving your vision, but you probably fear an operation on your eyes—especially after reading about a poor outcome in the popular press. Knowing the right questions to ask can help you achieve your goals and reduce your anxiety. Of course, caution is always prudent. But after performing tens of thousands of LASIK surgeries, I believe that patient education is the key to managing the fear of refractive surgery.

Such knowledge should enable you to use this sophisticated medical technology to your benefit. By following Karen through her exhaustive eye exam, her live LASIK surgery, and her short- and long-term recovery, you will gain a better understanding of what it's like to be a LASIK patient.

After reading this book you should begin to think more as an expert does. You will gain a better understanding of how your remarkable eyes work. You will have more insight into the benefits and risks of the operations mentioned earlier. You will know key questions to ask your doctor to see if you are a good candidate for refractive surgery. My goal in writing every chapter is to help you make an informed decision about your eyes. Only then can you decide if the benefits are worth the risks, considering your lifestyle. Do you want to have refractive surgery? Which kind? Are you a good candidate? If so, which procedure is right for you? And of paramount importance to your future vision, who should be your doctor?

Stephen Glenn Slade, M.D., FACS

INTRODUCTION

*You are creatures of light, we read. From light have you
come, to light shall you go, and surrounding you
through every step is the light of your infinite being.*
—Richard Bach, *One*

*An extremely nearsighted person, I was scheduled to have refractive
eye surgery to improve my vision in one week. Sitting in my garden in
the late afternoon, I squinted at the fuzzy image of my Boston fern
hanging on a limb of an enormous oak tree. I could barely see the
Monarch butterfly resting on an unfurling frond. Covered with
enzyme deposits, my soft disposable contacts—new only two hours
ago—failed to correct all of my nearsightedness and none of my astigmatism. I removed them. The butterfly—which hadn't moved—
faded from my view, and the fern became an amorphous green blob.*

*Filled with hopeful anticipation, I longed to know how well I
would be able to see my lovely garden after eye surgery. I reached into
my purse, grabbed my thick-edged glasses, and stared wistfully
through them at the fern and its splendid winged companion. Even in
the bright sunlight, the butterfly's vivid color now seemed dull, and*

the chartreuse new growth of my fern appeared much more blurred and several shades darker with glasses than with contacts. Unable to view my surroundings clearly, I turned inward, put my head on the table, and tried to fall asleep, hoping to free myself of anxiety.

Karen

Like my patient, Karen, about a quarter of the world's population is unable to see well without corrective lenses. To begin to understand why, let's follow a glorious streak of sunlight as it bounces off Karen's ethereal guest, the butterfly, and penetrates the amazing structures of your eye. Designed to focus light so that you can see clearly, your eye works rather like a camera.

Traveling at 186,000 miles per second, one brilliant bolt of light from the sun strikes the Monarch's gossamer wings, washing them with color. Determined to create a marvelous image for you, the reflected light rays are about to stream through your eye's dome-like window called the "cornea" (see figs. 1 and 2). Your primary light-focusing lens, your cornea is set in the leather-soft white of your eye, rather as a clear crystal is locked in a watch. Covering one-sixth of your eyeball, your oval cornea, which is only about one fiftieth of an inch thick, shields the inner workings of your optical system from the dangerous outside world.

A powerful *fixed* lens that refracts light, your cornea can be surgically reshaped to help you see nature's diaphanous "winged flower." A change of one one-hundredth of an inch (fifty microns) in the thickness of this transparent curved lens can easily make the difference between legal blindness and excellent sight. Not a simple structure that merely protects your eye, your corneal lens concentrates, or *bends*, light inward to focus the butterfly's image on the receptors of your "retina" (see figs. 1 and 5a). Hugging the back of the inside of your eyeball, your multi-layered retina—rather like

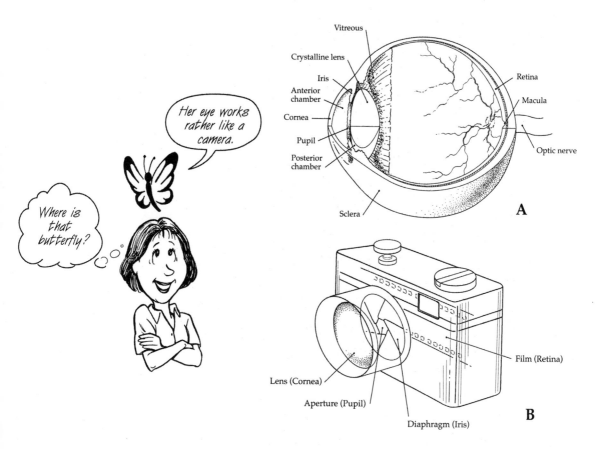

Figure 1

The human eye is often compared to a camera: Rather as the lenses of a camera focus images on film, the two lenses of the eye—the "cornea" (the clear fixed window of the eye) and the elastic "crystalline lens" (the adjustable lens inside the eye)—focus images on the "retina." The "pupil" is comparable to the camera's aperture and the "iris" relates to the diaphragm.

Note: The transparent dome-shaped cornea—the eye's most powerful light-focusing lens—is reshaped during excimer laser refractive surgery.

the film in a camera—is exquisitely sensitive to light. Composed of neurological tissue, your retina, which is designed to capture and transmit images, contains the "photoreceptors"—the "rods" and the "cones" that are named for their shape. Photochemically responsive to visual stimuli, they make up an important part of the light-gathering neural circuitry of your brain.

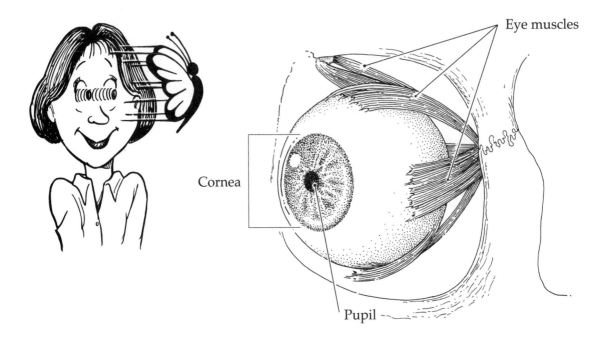

Figure 2
The six ocular muscles of the eye control the globe's split-second movements.

As the dazzling reflected light touches the tears that coat the outside of your cornea, its wet surface shines with the brilliance of a smooth polished jewel. This thin tear film covers your self-cleaning eye even when you aren't crying (see fig. 3). Bending the light rays ever so slightly inward toward your eye's dark entrance, known as the "pupil," your tears—which are vital to the health of your cornea—keep it supplied with dissolved oxygen from the air. With every blink of your eyelid, the watery three-layered tear film bathes your eye's window—which has no blood vessels—with oily lipids, dissolved salts, glucose, and mucus. Your tears act as a buffer against minor irritations such as smoke and fumes and contain an antibacterial enzyme that discourages infections. Since your cornea is richly supplied with nerves, the tiniest speck of dust will cause you to blink and tear.

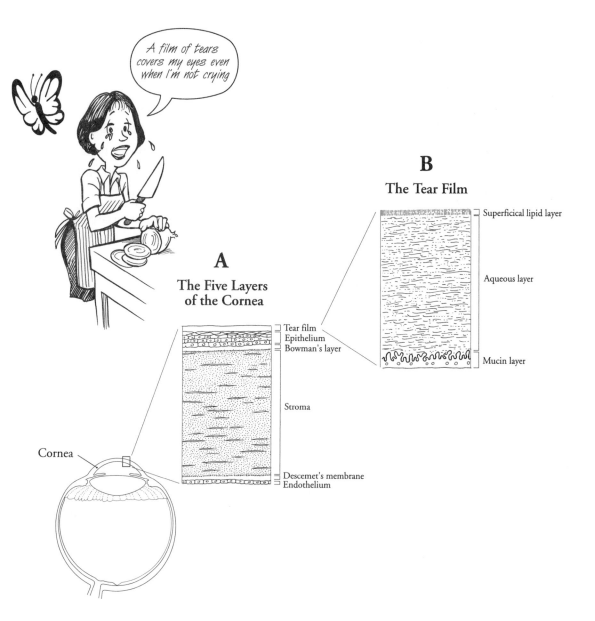

Figure 3

A. The five layers of the human cornea. The gel-like outer layer called the "epithelium," the second layer, or "Bowman's membrane," the middle layer called the "stroma," the fourth layer, or "Descemet's membrane," and the last layer, the cornea's metabolic pump, known as the "endothelium."

B. The tear film. A thin layer of tears lubricates the surface of the eye and provides vital oxygen and nutrients to the clear cornea, which has no blood vessels.

With its angle of attack slightly altered by your tears, the radiant sunlight rebounding from the Monarch now darts through each of the five crystal-clear layers of your cornea (see fig. 3). Only about five to seven cells thick, the outermost protective surface of your fixed lens, called the "epithelium" by doctors, helps guard your eye from dangerous invading microorganisms. Your epithelium possesses marvelous regenerative powers. Its cells are naturally replenished about every seven days.

When injured by a superficial, though excruciating, corneal abrasion, your epithelium will regenerate even more rapidly. If a twig gently brushes across your eye's gel-like epithelium, it will grow back without a scar in about one to three days. If the twig pierces the epithelium and injures one or both of the next two corneal layers, "Bowman's" layer and the "stroma," permanent scarring can occur. Unlike the epithelium, Bowman's thin membrane cannot regenerate. The epithelial cells bond to Bowman's unique smooth surface. Key to the outcome of the latest laser vision correction, the stroma, which makes up about 90 percent of the cornea's thickness, consists of layered, or "lamellar," collagen fibers. These lamellae, which are stacked in clear tiers rather like the layers of an onion, are specifically arranged in a geometrical design that allows the uninterrupted passage of the visible wavelengths of light. If the twig sharply cuts through the stroma beyond the final two corneal sections known as "Descemet's membrane" and the "endothelium"—fluid can leak from the interior of the eye, causing a drop in pressure and exposing the inner eye to infectious microorganisms.

Without the metabolic pumping action of your corneal endothelium, you would be unable to see your beautiful garden. A *single* layer of flat hexagonal cells, your eye's endothelium helps control the water-content of your cornea—which must be kept in a partially dehydrated state for crisp vision. Decreasing in number with age, these cells are unable to replace themselves and must increase in size to cover a damaged area. If endothelial cell count falls below a critical level, the cornea swells with excess fluid, resulting in a loss of transparency. When the cornea swells over the pupil, a distinct image cannot reach the retina.

Continuing along their journey through your gem-like eye, the intense light rays—which now have been refracted, or bent inward, by your corneal lens—stream through your pupil into your delicate inner eye. The size of your pupil's dark "opening" is controlled by your colored "iris" rather as the f/stop, or aperture, of a camera is governed by the action of its diaphragm (see fig. 1). A double muscle, your doughnut-shaped iris automatically expands and contracts like a pleated accordion to regulate the amount of light striking your retina. The color of your iris determines whether your eyes are blue, brown, green, or hazel. Since you are outside on a sunny day, your pupil constricts to almost pinpoint size to protect your sensitive photoreceptors from too much light stimulation.

Racing between the cornea and the iris, the light rays now penetrate a clear watery liquid called the "aqueous humor." This fluid circulates in the front chambers of the eye, flowing through the "anterior chamber" (see figs. 1 and 4). Supplying vital nourishment to the lenses of your eye, this clear watery liquid—which is continuously replenished and drained from the eye's front cavity—is under a relatively constant pressure. A dynamic force, the "intra-ocular pressure" stabilizes when liquid drainage equals fluid production. If the liquid that nourishes the lenses fails to drain properly, the pressure within the eye can become too high. When this potentially dangerous condition remains untreated, the optic nerve that carries visual information to the brain can be damaged, leading to a disease called glaucoma.

Before you can see close objects, the light must be focused by another lens inside your eye called the "crystalline lens" (see figs.

1 and 4). You may be familiar with how the lenses of a camera produce a well-defined photograph by changing the distance between the lenses and the film. Far more refined than any mechanical device, your flexible lens fine-tunes your vision by instantaneously changing shape to focus light. Suspended directly behind your fixed corneal lens and your iris by fine string-like ligaments called "zonular fibers," your adjustable lens provides about one-third of the light-bending power of your eye. Your amazing crystalline lens, which is the size and shape of a piece of M&M's candy, but about two-thirds water, allows your eye to refocus instantly when you are young. As you glance from the distant fern to your nearby hand, this pliable lens—which can "accommodate," or change shape, becoming rounder—works to place close images on your retina. Adding more power to your focusing system, your crystalline lens thickens when special "ciliary" muscles inside your eye release tension on the zonular fibers that control the shape of your lens.

As we age, this lens gradually loses its flexibility and thus its focusing ability, leading to a condition called "presbyopia," which literally means "old eyes." After age forty or so, even otherwise normally-sighted people begin to have problems seeing the fine print of a phone book. Eventually the newspaper becomes blurred, and reading glasses or bifocals are necessary. With time—at around age fifty-five, depending on the individual—the lens loses much of its ability to accommodate.

Remember when your grandmother needed cataract surgery because her vision was poor? Around age sixty or older the crystalline lens, which is surrounded by a clear elastic capsule, may become cloudy (see fig. 4). Examining the eyes with a special ophthalmic "slit-lamp" microscope, a doctor may see a noticeable light-filtering lens opacity called a cataract. It can become so dense that it blocks light's path to the retina. When the cataract interferes

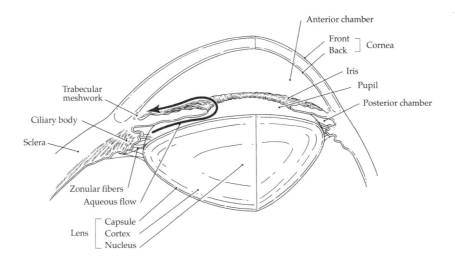

Figure 4

The front chambers of the eye (the "anterior" and "posterior chambers") and the crystalline lens inside the eye. Located behind the iris, the youthful crystalline lens changes shape to focus close objects. (During cataract surgery, a clouded lens can be removed and replaced with an artificial intra-ocular lens [IOL] implant.) Note how the lens sits in a skin-like capsule.

with the person's daily life, a surgeon can remove the clouded lens and replace it with an artificial "intra-ocular lens." Since this artificial lens has no ability to change shape, patients who have had cataract surgery wear reading glasses to focus up close.

Proceeding on the wondrous journey through your eye's delicate structures, the beam of light now penetrates the largest chamber of the eyeball. This dark space, pierced only by luminous images coming into focus, is filled with a transparent, jelly-like substance, the "vitreous humor" (see fig. 1). A relatively inert fluid, the vitreous helps hold your eye in its spherical shape. Although this viscous liquid is almost 99 percent water, it also contains hyaluronic acid—a natural shock absorber to help protect your retina from fast moving curveballs.

At last, the sun's speeding photons of light reflected off the butterfly approach your fragile retina. The self-restoring "videotape" of your living "TV camera," your retina is the most forward part of the nerve fibers of your brain. If you are nearsighted, or "myopic," like Karen, the particles of light will come to a focus in front of this wet, thin tissue, producing a fuzzy image of distant objects (see fig. 5c). If you are farsighted, or "hyperopic," the rays will reach a theoretical focal point behind your retinal curtain, forming an unclear picture (see fig. 5b). If you have "astigmatism," your central cornea is probably shaped like a football halved the long way rather than a basketball similarly cut. Since the astigmatic cornea is aspherical, the light rays are unequally bent. This means that they fail to meet at one point so that your eyesight is blurred at every distance (see fig. 5d). For those of you who are blessed with normal vision, the light will splash directly on your retinal receptors (see fig. 5a). Nevertheless, even if you have 20/20 vision, you will really never "see" the actual Monarch stroking the air. You will only sense its presence through the shafts of light that the butterfly's wings reflect.

Intent on completing their mission, the light rays carrying the Monarch's ever-changing image place it upside-down on the inside of the back of your eyeball. Capable of absorbing light, your retina's rods and cones—the photoreceptors, or nerve cells, named for their shape—convert the light energy into electrical signals that are relayed to your brain through your "optic nerve" (see fig. 1). Early in life, your clever brain learned to turn this flat inverted picture into a three-dimensional, right-side up image. Trained during infancy, your brain interprets the Monarch's coded message, allowing you to perceive far more than an insect attached to a plant. For you, the moving fingers of light paint a colored, animated work of art, a thing of beauty swaying in the soft breeze.

In order for you to discern the brilliant orange hues of the Monarch's wings, the three basic types of color-distinguishing pigments in your retinal cones must absorb the light rays.

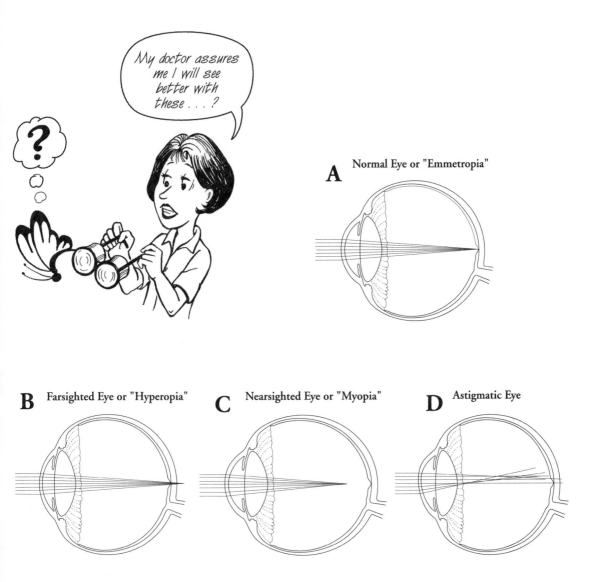

Figure 5

The emmetropic eye (A) has no refractive error. Defects in the focusing mechanism of the eye cause refractive errors. A person has a refractive error when the eye's two lenses fail to focus the image directly on to the retina, as in the most common refractive errors, hyperopia (B), myopia (C), and astigmatism (D).

A. The **normal** (emmetropic) eye focuses light directly on the retina for clear vision.

B. The **farsighted** (hyperopic) eye focuses light behind the retina.

C. The **nearsighted** (myopic) eye focuses light in front of the retina.

D. The **astigmatic** eye fails to focus light rays to a point, producing blurred images at every distance.

Concentrated near the center of your retina in a tiny indented area called the "fovea," the three kinds of cones, which each respond to a specific light wave, enable you to discern red, blue, and green—light's primary colors (see figs. 1 and 6). The cones normally provide your most detailed vision in good light. Your "visual axis" is an imaginary line drawn from a viewed object through your pupil to your fovea (see fig. 6). Your sight-giving fovea, which contains no rods, is located in the middle of the round "macula" of the retina. Called "macular degeneration," deterioration of the irreplaceable, cone-rich macula in some older people causes a degradation of straight-ahead vision. Most people can discern several hundred colors within the visible spectrum of light. Some partially color-blind patients, however, have a hereditary disorder of the pigments in their cones and are unable to distinguish some shades. Few people are totally color-blind.

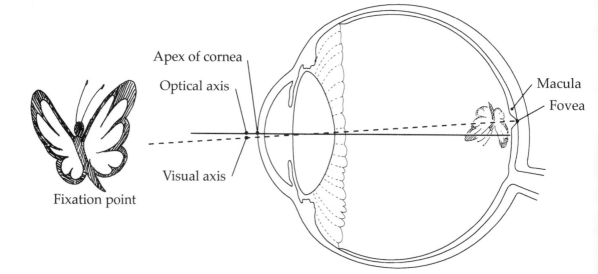

Figure 6

The "visual axis" or line-of-sight connects the object of regard with the "fovea," the area of the retina that provides the most acute vision. Located inside the back of the globe of the eye (the "fundus") in the middle of the irreplaceable "macula," the fovea is a tiny indented area rich in the light-sensitive photoreceptors called the "cones."

Your versatile eyes give you the irreplaceable gift of sight in bright sunlight and in dim starlight—from a sunny beach to a moonlit one. When you first enter a movie theater, your eyes need time to adjust to the dark. The pigment in your retinal rods, known as "rhodopsin," consists of a vitamin A-like chemical compound and a protein. Called "visual purple," this pigment absorbs light and helps you see in semi-darkness, producing black and white images and all the shades of gray. As they strike the retina, light rays bleach out the rhodopsin in your rods, generating electrical signals. These are transmitted to the brain's visual cortex in the back of your head via a bundle of fibers that make up the optic nerve. The light-induced changes in the chemical structure of vitamin A must be reversed in order for you to see in low light conditions. The complete renewal of the visual pigment takes about ten to thirty minutes. Without your rods, you would suffer from night-blindness.

As you admire your garden, your eyes work together to help you perceive the distance between you and the fern. Each of your eyes views the Monarch from a somewhat different angle, producing a slightly dissimilar image on each of your retinas. Since the muscles of your two eyes keep both of your retinal foveae pointed at one spot, your brain is able to fuse the images, providing you with "binocular vision" and depth perception. In a way, the two visual representations of the Monarch overlap and produce one mental image. This effect is easier to fathom if you think of how your brain fuses each eye's separate view when you look at a football field through binoculars, although of course natural vision isn't magnified. Only through the balanced muscle coordination of your two eyes, can you enjoy "stereoscopic" vision and acute three-dimensional depth perception.

Once the electrical impulses from your retinas are parsed and magically "reassembled" by your brain, you become conscious of the dainty, sunlit creature perched on your fern. Through the complex physiological process of vision, not only do you recognize the Monarch's familiar shape, but you behold the beauty of the slow, easy motion of its translucent wings. With each sweep of the butterfly's graceful appendages, subtle, ever-changing hues of vibrant oranges and soft, rich browns flood your gaze. Through your superb eyes, you embrace the form, color, depth, texture, and movement of your lovely visitor. Suddenly, for one fleeting instant—a visual keepsake forever burned into your memory— you feel the wonder of the mystery and miracle of sight. Leaving no permanent trace of their presence on your eyes, the rays of sunlight have fulfilled their destiny. Through them, you and your elusive guest are at one with your garden—if only for a moment.

CHAPTER One

WHAT CAN CORNEAL REFRACTIVE EYE SURGERY DO FOR YOU?

The ancient Greeks explained the mystery of sight by declaring that perception occurs when "internal fire" from the eye mixes with "external fire" from an object.
— "The Sense of Sight," National Geographic

It was a fresh spring morning. I had awakened early because a robin outside my bedroom was chirping away in wild abandon. Carefully removing my clear plastic eye patch, I glanced at my digital clock, which was about to start buzzing. No longer a total blur, the inch-high numbers on its face were now in focus. Without the aid of glasses for nearsightedness, I silenced the alarm, jumped out of bed, and flung open my second story window. Taking a deep breath of the heavy, gloriously scented air, I gazed at my Formosa azaleas. Covered with dark pink buds, they were about to burst into bloom. I turned and bounded across my bedroom toward the bathroom door and, for once, didn't run into my coffee table.

Looking in the mirror, I clearly beheld my unmade face without thick-edged glasses for the first time in my adult life. What a shock. Although my curly dark hair was standing on end, my eyes sparkled, and my cheeks were rosy. Slowly, a huge unstoppable grin spread from one ear to the other. I look healthy, I thought. No one would ever guess that I had eye surgery recently. After examining my teeth, I reached for my toothpaste. With surprise, I noticed that I could read the label without holding it two inches from my nose. Another small pleasure.

As I turned on the shower, I discovered that I could see the soap dish. Even the water marks on the glass door didn't bother me. That morning—two days after my eye surgery—was the beginning of one of the happiest days of my life. I could see! Not only could I see the coat hangers in my closet, but I could see my bright yellow egg on my breakfast plate.

As I drove down the street without glasses, I waved at my neighbor. Approaching the feeder road, I noted the intense color of the red stop light. More sure of my vision—and thus my ability to react—the cars flying by on the freeway were less frightening than before my operation. I opened my sunroof and pushed the accelerator almost to the floor. Like a hummingbird let out of a dim covered cage, I was free. I felt like the luckiest person in the world. But the truth was—luck had nothing to do with my miraculous new eyesight. Over fifty years of dedicated determination on the part of hundreds of people had changed my life.

Karen

THE ELUSIVE DREAM OF PERFECT VISION

The eye has a passion to see. Forty percent of the input to your brain comes from your eyes. Your vision affects every aspect of your life. Through your sight, you behold the flutter of a butterfly wing, the icy chill of a confidant's betrayal, and the adoration in your lover's smile. Penetrating your mind like a swift sword, a single image can unleash a cascade of shattering emotions. In the batting of an eye, a compelling look has weakened the mightiest will, commanding its total surrender. Focused shafts of light, amplified by your retina and interpreted by your brain, can trigger a complex series of chemical reactions within your body. Turning up the heat, adrenaline quickens your pulse. Your heart pumps primal hormonal messages throughout your bloodstream. Capable of igniting love at first sight, a mere glance can break your vulnerable heart or steal it for a lifetime. Only with your eyes, can you completely capture the moment. If you miss the magic, it is gone in an instant, never to return.

If you are nearsighted or farsighted, you may fantasize about waking up in the morning able to see the landscapes of your world without glasses or contact lenses. Like Karen, you probably yearn to have clear, comfortable, binocular vision without sticking something in or in front of your eyes. The simple pleasures of keen eyesight that many people take for granted elude your gaze.

Today, the realization of a long-awaited goal—the dream of relatively accurate unaided vision—is now possible by surgically treating the eye. At last, modern medical technology is able to answer the prayer for reduced dependence on corrective lenses for nearsightedness, farsightedness, and astigmatism (see fig. 7). As much an art as a science, an amazing new refractive eye operation that can now refocus your eyes is changing lives forever. By harnessing the power of today's sophisticated computers and the remarkable precision of the laser, a specially trained ophthalmologist can improve your vision without glasses. Looking at the surgical field through the high magnification of a microscope, a refractive surgeon can reshape your cornea—the transparent window of the eye—using a cool, invisible light scalpel called an excimer, or crystal, laser. The difference of a tiny fraction of a millimeter in the steepness of this corneal lens can dramatically improve the quality of your life. By bringing shimmering oak leaves, pink rose petals, and your child's angelic face into more perfect view, better vision can set you free to take in the world around you.

A. The Nearsighted Eye

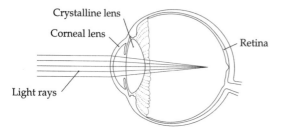

B. The Farsighted Eye

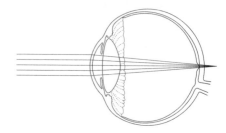

Concave Lens to Focus a Nearsighted Eye

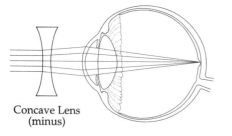

Concave Lens
(minus)

Convex Lens to Focus a Farsighted Eye

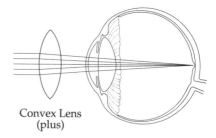

Convex Lens
(plus)

C. Normally-Focused Eye

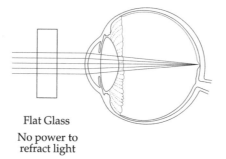

Flat Glass

No power to
refract light

Figure 7

A. A minus, or concave, lens corrects, nearsightedness. A minus lens, which subtracts power from the eye's optical system, "pre-spreads" light, causing the rays of light to diverge before they enter the cornea. A minus lens moves the focal point of the image from in front of the retina backward onto it.

B. A plus, or convex, lens corrects farsightedness and age-related presbyopia. A plus lens, which adds power to the eye's optical system, bends light rays, causing them to converge before they enter the cornea. A plus lens "pulls" the theoretical focal point of the image from behind the retina forward onto it.

C. Not a lens, a flat piece of glass with parallel sides is unable to bend light.

As the history of vision correction surgery shows, realizing the dream of clear, unaided eyesight has never been easy. When most people think of refractive surgery to refocus the eye, they think of "radial keratotomy," or RK—the first operation to correct nearsightedness. This procedure, which was brought from Russia to the U.S. in the late 1970s, is not laser-based. The surgeon attempts to improve his patient's vision by cutting spoke-like radial incisions in the cornea with a guarded diamond-tipped knife (see fig. 8). The tiny slits are invisible to the naked eye. Although RK has helped many patients, this surgery, as we discuss in detail later, has limitations.

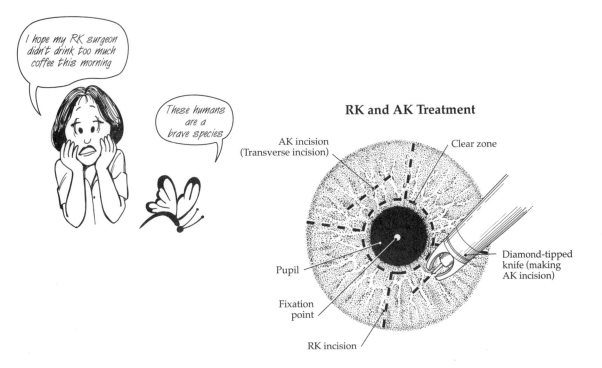

Figure 8

RK or "radial keratotomy." A non-laser-based refractive procedure, RK was the first elective operation to reduce nearsightedness. Using a guarded diamond-tipped knife, the surgeon makes spoke-like radial incisions in the cornea to flatten its surface.

AK or "astigmatic keratotomy." During a surgical technique known as astigmatic keratotomy, the doctor places transverse and arcuate (curved incisions) in the cornea to treat astigmatism.

Surgeons performed the first laser-based procedure in the late 1980s. After extensive clinical trials, ophthalmologists looked with great hope to the cool new excimer laser to provide patients with rapid, predictable results. But, unfortunately, the original operation, called "PRK" (photorefractive keratectomy), has failed to live up to many doctors' early expectations. During this procedure, surgeons remove the thin, gel-like outer corneal layer called the epithelium. Laser pulses are aimed at the newly exposed surface of the cornea to vaporize microscopic layers of tissue, thereby changing the curvature of the eye's transparent outer lens (see fig. 9). Although many mildly and moderately nearsighted patients have been helped by this operation, for reasons we will discuss in detail later, PRK patients sometimes hesitate to recommend it to their friends.

Throughout this book, we refer to focusing errors as "mild," "moderate," and "severe," based on "diopters," a measurement unit used to quantify the light-bending power of a lens. Diopters define the exact amount of correction you need. A 1 diopter lens can bring light rays to a focus one meter away from the lens. So if you have a -1 diopter lens prescription (written as -1D), your eye focuses clearly without correction at one meter, or approximately the length of your arm. If you need a-2 diopter lens, which is twice as strong, you can focus light at only half a meter. This means that you can see clearly without glasses about half way down your arm. If you need a-10 diopter lens, your eye focuses light at about two inches from your nose. We sometimes tell patients to think of diopters in relative terms; the more out of focus the eye, the higher the number used to represent the refractive error. For a further explanation see insert 1, *What Are "Diopters"?* on page 22 and insert 2, *Measuring Visual Acuity: What Is 20/20, or "Normal," Eyesight?* on page 23 (see the Snellen eye chart in fig. 10).

PRK Laser Treatment

Removal of the Eye's Outer Coating

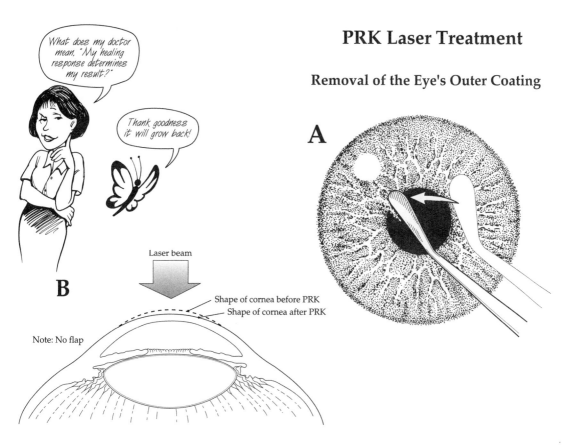

A

B

Laser beam

Shape of cornea before PRK
Shape of cornea after PRK

Note: No flap

What does my doctor mean, "My healing response determines my result?"

Thank goodness it will grow back!

Re-growth of Eye's Outer Gel-like Coating

C

Day 1: 30% healed   Day 2: 70% healed   Day 3: 100% healed

Figure 9

PRK or "photorefractive keratectomy." An excimer laser-based refractive surface procedure to reduce mild and moderate nearsightedness.

A. Removing the gel-like coating of the cornea called the "epithelium."

B. A microsurgeon uses a computer-controlled laser to flatten the curvature of the cornea. Note: No protective tissue flap covers the exposed wound.

C. The re-growth of the coating of the cornea of the eye, the epithelium, usually takes about three days, but healing continues for months.

INSERT 1

WHAT ARE "DIOPTERS"?

To write your glasses or contact lens prescription, your doctor must determine your exact refractive error. Your correction is expressed in diopters that measure how much a corrective lens must bend light to focus it on your retina to normalize your vision. A lens that can *bend* parallel light rays to a focal point of 1 meter is said to have a power of 1 diopter (1.00D). A 2-diopter lens can focus light rays at a point 0.5 meters away from itself.

If you are blessed with normal eyesight, your eye doctor will write in your chart that your "sphere" is 0.0D, or "plano" (pl). This means, of course, that you have no refractive error. Department store sunglasses without power are plano lenses. *Only curved surfaces bend light; flat surfaces do not.*

If you have a myopic correction of -1 diopter, you are focused at 1 meter, or approximately the length of your arm. Without glasses, objects farther away than your hand will be slightly blurred and will become progressively more indistinct the further in the distance you look. With this refractive error, and no other visual defects, you should be able to read most street signs in good light. If your refraction is - 2 diopters, you are focused at 0.5 meters, and you can only see clearly halfway down your arm. With this refractive error, you dare not drive without glasses. Nonetheless, you can see better in the distance than a person who is more nearsighted—someone, for example, whose correction is -3 diopters.

If you are farsighted, your amount of correction is expressed in positive numbers (+1 diopter of hyperopia, e.g.).

With nearsightedness, a refractive or focusing error less than -5 diopters is considered mild "myopia." Myopia is the medical term for nearsightedness and is corrected with a "minus" lens. Five to 7 or 8 diopters is in the moderate range, and greater than 7 or 8 is

INSERT 2

MEASURING VISUAL ACUITY: WHAT IS
20/20, OR "NORMAL," EYESIGHT?

You probably remember reading the big *E* on your doctor's Snellen eye chart at your last appointment. Many people confuse their eyeglasses prescription, which is measured in diopters, with their eye chart readings, which assess visual acuity (VA). By ascertaining the smallest line of figures that you can distinguish at a specified distance, your physician can determine your VA. If you can read the 20/20 line at 20 feet (about 6 meters), your visual acuity equals 20/20 (or 6/6 in meters), which is normal. If you read the 20/40 line at 20 feet, you see at 20 feet what the normally-sighted person sees at 40 feet.

Your VA, as measured by the Snellen eye chart, cannot be accurately converted to diopters. Nonetheless, assuming that your eyes are healthy, and you have no refractive error affecting distance vision, you should be able to read the 20/20 line or better. If your myopic refraction is -1 diopter, you should be able to read the 20/40 or 20/50 line of the eye chart. If you have significant astigmatism, however, you probably wouldn't have 20/20 visual acuity. In addition, if your eye has some underlying pathology—even though light is perfectly focused on your retina—you may be unable to read the 20/20 line.

called severe. About 90 percent of nearsighted people have a refractive error of less than -6 diopters. Only about one nearsighted person in ten has severe myopia. Nevertheless, even if you have only -4 diopters of nearsightedness, you may feel that your correction is severe because you are almost totally dependent on your glasses or contact lenses. With astigmatism, less than 1 diopter is considered mild. One to 2 diopters is moderate. Two to 3 diopters is severe, and greater than 3 diopters is extreme. With farsightedness, greater than +5 diopters is called severe "hyperopia," the medical term for farsightedness. This refractive error is corrected with a "plus" lens. See insert 3, *Reading Your Eyeglasses Prescription, on page 25.*

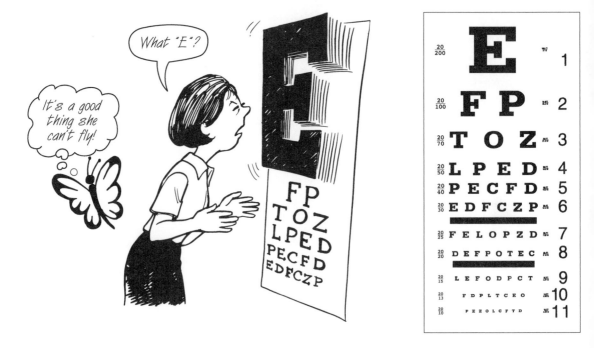

Figure 10
The Snellen eye chart to measure visual acuity.

Now, after years of research, ophthalmologists finally have a "patient friendly" procedure that, in exquisitely skilled hands, delivers excellent, relatively stable results in a more elegant fashion than the older refractive operations. Known as LASIK (an acronym for *las*er *in* situ *k*eratomileusis), this new excimer laser outpatient procedure is one of the first operations in the history of medicine to use a computer-driven light scalpel to reshape part of the human body. The Greek word *keratomileusis* is literally translated as "carving of the cornea." (*Kerato* means "cornea" and *mileusis* means "carving.") During LASIK, an ophthalmologist uses an

Insert 3
Reading Your Eyeglasses
Prescription

When your eye doctor hands you a prescription for glasses or contact lenses to correct nearsightedness, farsightedness, astigmatism, or age-related presbyopia, how do you read the esoteric notation? As you know, your prescription, which is measured in diopters, is the power that must be put in each corrective lens to *counteract* your refractive error in the respective eye. Your prescription is expressed with the following formula:

Sphere (D) + or - Cylinder Power (D) @ Cylinder Axis
(in degrees)

This simply means that if you have -3 diopters of nearsightedness in your right eye and -3.5 diopters of myopia in your left eye—and no astigmatism—your glasses prescription might read:

O.D. (right eye) - 3.00(D) and O.S. (left eye) -3.50(D)

If you also have 0.25 diopters of *myopic* astigmatism in your left eye, your prescription may read:

O.S. -3.50(D) -0.25(D) @ 180 degrees axis.

This means that to correct your left eye (O.S.) you need a minus (concave) -3.5 spherical lens combined with a -0.25 cylindrical lens at an axis of 180 degrees. Since the axis is at 180 degrees, the astigmatism is horizontal. By looking at this glasses prescription, your doctor knows that both meridians of your cornea bend light too much: the *flattest meridian* refracts light short of the retina by 3.5 diopters, and the steepest one by 3.75 diopters. Put another way, with this prescription, you would have -3.5 diopters of myopia combined with -0.25 cylinder astigmatism. If you also need bifocal correction for age-related presbyopia, your doctor might write:

Add = +1.50(D)

continued

READING YOUR EYEGLASSES
PRESCRIPTION (CONTINUED)

This means that you need +1.5 diopters more plus power in the lower portion of your glasses to help you focus to read. Added algebraically to the -3.5 diopter prescription of your left lens, the power in your bifocal prescription in that eye would be:

-2.00D (-3.50D plus +1.50D equals -2.00D).

electromechanically controlled surgical blade to cut a round "hinged" flap from the surface of the anesthetized cornea, the eye's curved window (see fig. 11). Leaving one uncut edge of the protective flap attached to the eye, the doctor carefully folds back this thin tissue, exposing the delicate inner corneal layer called the stroma (see fig. 3). To correct myopia, he then aims the cool, ultraviolet laser directly over the light-gathering pupil to remove microscopic layers of corneal tissue. For most nearsighted patients, the laser beam is concentrated on the eye only ten or twenty seconds, although larger refractive errors require more treatment. After the cornea's curvature is thus remodeled, the physician gently puts the living flap back in place. No stitches are necessary. (See chapter 2 for a detailed description of this operation.)

The results depend on the patient's eyes and healing response, the doctor's skill, and the laser. One study involving thousands of patients using the broad beam Summit Apex Plus and the VISX Star showed good results at three months after LASIK surgery. With the Summit, about 50 percent of mildly and moderately nearsighted eyes up to -7 diopters achieved 20/20 on the Snellen eye chart or better without glasses, (see eye chart in fig. 10). Approximately 93 percent of nearsighted eyes with corrections between -8 and -14 diopters achieved 20/40 or better. With the

VISX Star, over 54 percent of patients with corrections up to -7 diopters achieved 20/20 or better. Almost 95 percent of patients between -8 and -14 diopters achieved 20/40 or better.

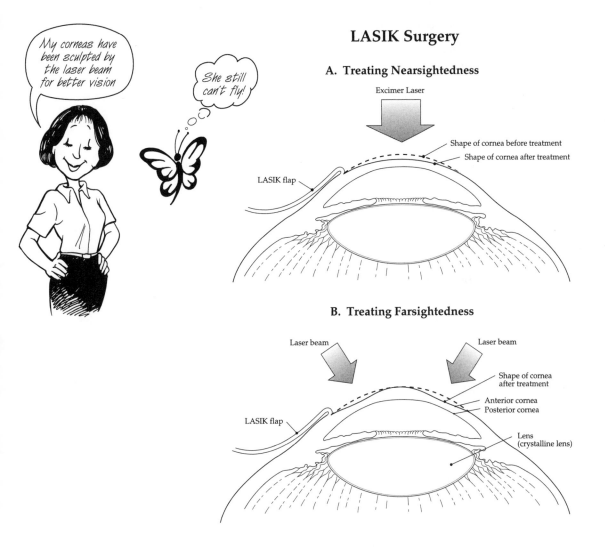

LASIK Surgery

A. Treating Nearsightedness

B. Treating Farsightedness

Figure 11

A. Excimer laser surgery for *nearsightedness* changes the shape of the window of the eye, flattening the powerful corneal lens to improve visual acuity.

B. Excimer laser surgery for *farsightedness* has a steepening effect on the basic shape of the corneal lens. Notice the "anterior" (front) surface of the cornea and the "posterior" (back) of the cornea. Both refract light.

All laser companies, including Summit and VISX, continuously strive to upgrade their machines. One smaller study using a new, fast-scanning laser, the Bausch & Lomb Technolas 217, found that following LASIK surgery by *experienced* doctors, 99.7 percent of *mildly* and *moderately* nearsighted patients could read the 20/40 line or better on the eye chart without corrective lenses, and 87.3 percent achieved normal 20/20 vision or better.

Nearly eliminating the inflammatory wound-healing response common to other refractive procedures, this stealth-like surgical technique—whose effects are invisible to the naked eye—is easy on the patient, causing minimal discomfort during and after this short operation. Most patients have rapid initial return to vision. They often see remarkably well immediately after this procedure. Many people return to work the next day, although severely nearsighted persons, those with dry eyes, and older folks have a slower recovery. The majority of patients attain their final outcome in about three months.

By greatly improving vision, LASIK can profoundly transform people's lives, awakening a new sense of awareness on many levels. Whatever the pre-surgical refractive error, six months or a year after LASIK, patients often say they have undergone a significant lifestyle change because they can see better. Some people seem to approach their daily lives with renewed enthusiasm. Depending on their post-surgical outcome, many patients are able to conduct their normal activities without correction, although some individuals still need thin glasses or contact lenses. Improved vision enables people to interact more effectively with their environment.

Contact lenses also have changed many lives, but not everyone can wear them. Some people have a problem inserting contacts in their eyes. A few patients have an immune response to having foreign objects resting on their corneas. Others become contact-lens intolerant as they get older. At first they may experience minor eye irritations that contribute to increasingly longer periods of contact lens down-time. Uncomfortable with lenses, persons with dry eyes—many of whom are baby boomers—want to be less dependent on corrective lenses. People who are concerned because their contact lenses cause repeated bacterial or viral eye infections might wish to consider refractive surgery. Some patients are forced to give up contacts because they can cause "neovascularization" of the cornea, a condition in which tiny blood vessels grow into the cornea. If these become severe, they can obscure vision. Patients who are free of contacts say that a significant cause of stress—eye pain—has been removed from their lives. Able to move their eyes around with ease, such patients can connect visually and emotionally with others. Some even become more self-confident, outgoing, and friendly.

The joys of good vision without corrective lenses are expressed differently depending on the patient's interests and concerns. Pete, a twenty-seven-year-old attorney, likes to race sail boats. "It is so great," he said, "not to worry about dust getting under my contacts or the wind popping a lens out of my eye. I am an extremely active guy. I hated being continually dependent on contacts or spectacles. When my glasses weren't lost, they were broken" (see insert 4, *Your Non-surgical Options* on page 30).

Nancy, a young working mother of a baby girl, said: "My peripheral vision with spectacles was poor. When I was a child, the boys would come up along side of me and snatch my glasses and hide them. As an adult walking alone at night, I used to worry that someone would grab my spectacles—that I would be helpless. Since my surgery, I feel more in control—more able to take care of my little girl and myself on a trip or in an emergency."

Another patient with two-hundred-watt blue eyes said, "One of my co-workers implied that I am vain because I don't want to wear

Insert 4
Your Non-Surgical Options

Glasses

If the lenses of your eyes fail to focus images on your retinas, you have the option of wearing glasses or contact lenses to see well. As you know, glasses, which are the safest way to correct refractive errors, improve eyesight by putting a lens in front of the each eye. Spectacles for myopia refocus the light entering your eye with a *concave* lens (it bows inward) that is thinner in the middle than around the edges. Simply put, such a minus lens—which subtracts power from your optical system—"pre-spreads" the light, causing the rays of light to diverge before they enter your cornea (see fig. 5). A minus lens moves the focal point of an image from in front of the retina onto the photoreceptors of the retina.

Glasses and contact lenses correct farsightedness by refocusing the light that enters your eye with a *convex* lens (it bows outward) that is thicker in the middle than around the edges. Such a plus lens—which adds power to your optical system—"pre-bends" the light, causing the rays to converge more rapidly before they enter your cornea. A plus lens brings the focal point from behind your retina forward onto its photoreceptors (see fig. 5).

Contact Lenses

Contact lenses can correct eyesight by refocusing light through a clear, hard-milled or soft hydrophilic disk (one with a high water content) that floats on the surface of your eye. Like glasses, contacts for near- and farsightedness shift the focal point of light, placing images directly on each retina. Rigid gas-permeable lenses (RGPs), usually provide clearer, crisper vision than soft contact lenses (SCLs). By creating a

continued

YOUR NON-SURGICAL OPTIONS (CONTINUED)

spherical refracting surface, rigid lenses can correct not only near- and farsightedness, but also astigmatism. Many people, however, are unable to tolerate rigid lenses.

Most patients find SCLs more comfortable than RGPs, but SCLs—which mold to the surface of the eye—often fail to correct astigmatism. Even though specially-designed "toric" soft lenses correct astigmatism, not everyone can wear them. Allowing increased oxygen transmissibility, extended-wear soft contact lenses provide increased comfort and can be made to correct astigmatism. Disposable soft contacts, which many people cannot feel in their eyes, are extremely convenient because you can throw them away at the end of the day. Unfortunately, they fail to correct significant astigmatism.

Interestingly enough, sometimes even a soft lens without toric correction will mask up to 1 diopter of astigmatism, depending on the contact's ability to hold its shape. Some soft lenses are thicker than others. If a patient can wear a soft contact that has sufficient body, or "memory," even a spherical lens without toric correction may offset low amounts of astigmatism.

my glasses. She just doesn't realize that my spectacles—especially since the lenses are unusually thick—are a barrier between me and the rest of the world. When I wear my glasses at a company board meeting, I almost feel like a non-person. Even though I am an expert in my field, some people avoid eye contact with me, failing to acknowledge my presence. This almost never happens when I wear my contact lenses. When I was a shy teenager, I could almost hide behind my spectacles if I didn't feel like talking."

Some patients needlessly worry that refractive surgery will permanently change the appearance of their eyes. Without the aid of a special ophthalmic microscope, even your doctor will be unable to tell that you have had an eye operation (see fig. 12). Sometimes people confuse vision correction procedures with cosmetic surgery. Refractive surgery is not plastic surgery. Years ago doctors even debated whether RK was cosmetic surgery. You rarely hear surgeons discuss this anymore. Now, if someone has a face lift—yes, that is cosmetic surgery because it changes the person's looks. Although both operations are elective procedures, plastic surgery changes *form* while refractive surgery improves *function*. Laser surgery does have a cosmetic aspect because most patients look better without glasses, but these procedures in no way make the eye look different. If an orthopedic surgeon repairs a crippled woman's legs, is this

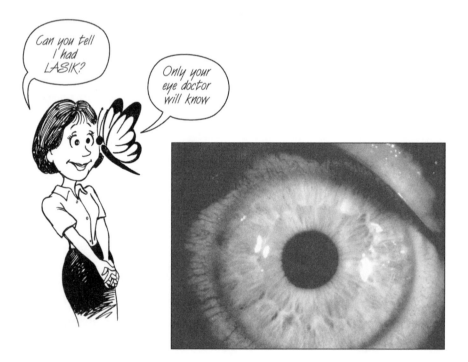

Figure 12

Once the eye heals, even an eye doctor without the aid of a special ophthalmic microscope is unable to tell that a patient has had refractive laser eye surgery. The slide above shows an excimer laser-treated eye one day after LASIK surgery.

operation cosmetic surgery because the woman doesn't have to be seen with crutches anymore? Of course not. By changing the way the eye *focuses*, excimer laser surgery allows patients to see better.

Vision correction surgery treats refractive errors, but it cannot make a blind eye see, a diseased eye healthy, or an old eye young. These operations do not treat glaucoma, cataracts, or retinal diseases. Even though you should see better after treatment, LASIK, PRK, and RK do not cure nearsightedness. A refractive surgeon can refocus nearsighted eyes, but they still will be classified as myopic. After surgery, your yearly eye examination will be as important as ever. Although the curvature of your cornea will be flatter, the length of your eyeball will remain unchanged. Later in life, the severely nearsighted eye is more likely to deteriorate than the normal eye. If you are extremely myopic, your eyeball may be elongated, and the retina at the back of each eye may be thinner than normal. Rather like wallpaper attached to an old shifting wall, the retina of an extremely nearsighted patient is stretched over an expanded surface. Such a patient might be more prone to retinal tears, holes, and detachments. In a condition called "myopic degeneration," the retina becomes so stretched that correctable visual acuity, or sharpness of vision, drops.

Refractive surgery does not slow the aging process. As the lens inside the eye ages, almost everyone becomes "presbyopic" and needs reading glasses or bifocals, even though nearsighted people can remove their glasses or contacts to see up close. When both eyes are surgically corrected for distance, reading glasses usually are necessary for older patients. In other words, the presbyopic nearsighted patient trades glasses to correct distance vision for magnifiers to focus near objects. As discussed in detail later, the good news is that some nearsighted surgery patients who have one eye corrected for distance and the other one left slightly undercorrected for close work may be able to drive and to read with little or no correction.

CORRECTING NEARSIGHTEDNESS

You will recall that if you are nearsighted or myopic, light is focused in front of your retina rather than on it (see fig. 5). Objects in the distance appear blurry. The further in front of the retina that light comes to a focal point, the progressively more blurred vision becomes. The nearsighted eyeball is too long from front to back for the lenses of the eye to focus light on the retina. (The axial length of your eye may be too long, or your cornea may be steeper than normal, or both). Since most patients with myopia can see close objects relatively clearly, this refractive error is called nearsightedness. More than 70 million people in North America are myopic.

To correct nearsightedness surgically, a highly skilled doctor uses the excimer laser to flatten the curvature of the powerful cornea—although its basic shape will still be convex (see fig. 11a). Depending on your age, your transparent, fixed corneal lens provides approximately two-thirds of your focusing power. During laser surgery, the ophthalmologist removes microscopic cells from the center of the dome-shaped cornea, creating a newly contoured living "lens" within the patient's own tissue. By changing the steepness of the window of your eye, surgery adjusts the refractive power of your cornea, making it a weaker lens for nearsightedness (rather like adding a minus lens with glasses). Ideally, after laser treatment, the nearsighted corneal lens will no longer be too steep and thus too powerful for the length of the eyeball. Since such a steep cornea bends light too much, the image is focused in front of the retina. Once correctly treated, the cornea can focus light on or closer to the retina so that vision is clearer.

MORE NATURAL VISION

Refractive surgery allows more comfortable natural-like vision. If you wear thick-edged glasses for nearsightedness, you probably have noticed that they make objects appear smaller. Looking through high-powered spectacles is rather like viewing the world through the wrong end of binoculars. The farther your corrective lenses are from your eyes, the smaller the image placed on your retinas. Eye doctors call this phenomenon the "minification" effect (see fig. 13). If you have switched from wearing glasses to contacts, you may have noticed a decrease in this minification effect because contacts are closer to your eyes. Refractive surgery for myopia further enlarges the image placed on your retina. Since the power of the corneal lens is surgically adjusted, one might say that the "correction" is put within the cornea, allowing more natural vision. For about every 7 diopters improvement in nearsightedness after surgery, minification is reduced enough to improve your best-corrected visual acuity by one line on the eye chart.

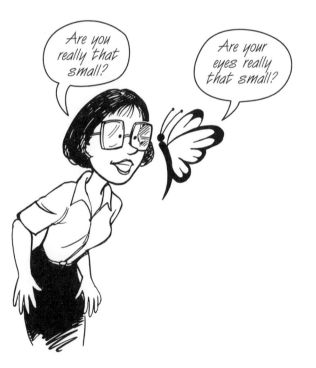

Figure 13

The "minification" effect. Thick-edged glasses for nearsightedness make objects appear smaller than normal. The more correction, the greater the minification effect.

Another important disadvantage of glasses is that they limit your peripheral vision. Even if you wear unobtrusive frames, glasses restrict your field of vision as you gaze across the horizon. They don't provide the "wrap-around" eyesight that contact lenses and refractive surgery do.

Strong glasses—which have highly curved lenses—not only interfere with peripheral vision, they also distort images because of a phenomenon known as "spherical aberration." If you have ever looked through a crystal ball or a round, glass snow globe, you may have noticed the effect of spherical aberration. You can see better through the center than through the edges. Light rays coming through either side near your face are bent progressively more than those coming through the center. The latter are parallel. The more the shafts of light are bent, the more they fall short of your retina, meaning that they fail to come to a focal point (see fig. 14). Similarly, glasses for severe myopia fail to focus bundles of light coming in through the edges at the same point as light coming through the center. Although modern lens-grinding techniques decrease the "fishbowl" effect of spherical aberration, glasses with large amounts of correction still can distort vision. By making you less dependent on glasses, refractive surgery can give you a more expansive outlook on the world.

If you have a significant difference in the refractive error between your two eyes, you may find glasses intolerable. In such a case, the most nearsighted eye puts a smaller image on its retina than the other eye. Hard as it may try, your brain cannot fuse a large dissimilarity in the sizes of the images falling on your retinas. Called "anisometropia" by eye doctors, this condition, which typically becomes a problem with a 2 diopters or greater difference between the eyes, can be corrected with either contact lenses or refractive surgery.

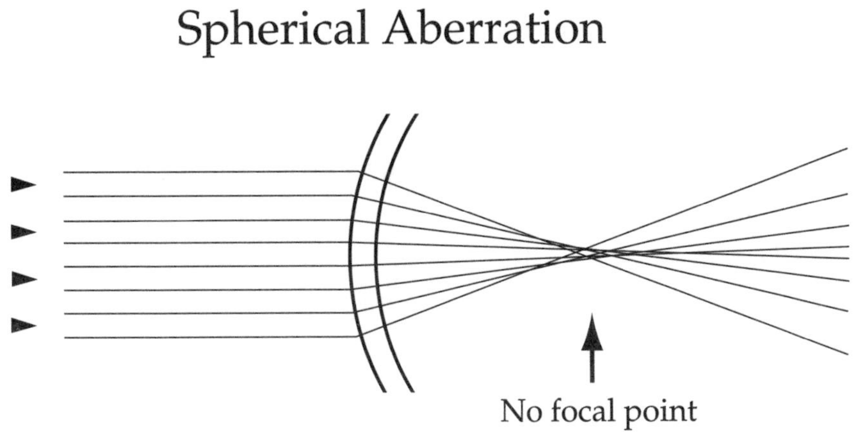

Spherical Aberration

No focal point

Figure 14

"Spherical aberration." A distortion of images that occurs with high-power lenses.

For example, glasses for severe nearsightedness fail to focus bundles of light coming in through the edges at the same point as light coming through the center.

Note: No focal point.

If you are nearsighted, you may have noticed that your night vision with glasses is less sharp than that of some of your friends. After refractive surgery, your eyes should be better focused in dim light, but these operations do not treat all the problems associated with severe myopia that cause "night-blindness." Even though many people do report improved low-light visual acuity following LASIK, some patients who have poor night vision before the operation may have the same complaint afterwards.

If you are nearsighted, you become even more so at night. In addition, if you have large pupils, you may have poorer night vision than someone with normal-size pupils. Why? To simplify a complicated concept, think how an expensive camera with its aperture wide-open loses focus more easily than a throw-away model with a small aperture. To let in more light, the eye's pupil dilates when illumination is low (see fig. 15). When your pupil opens in dim light, its diameter increases from approximately three millimeters to about six millimeters so that a bigger image falls on the retina. The larger the pupil, the more cornea you use. At night, a shadow-like ghosting effect can occur around street lamps because light rays are bent at different angles across the cornea. Since it is "aspheric," or unequally curved, the cornea has multiple refractive powers across its surface, along a radius from the center to the edge. Rigid gas permeable contact lenses, which allow more oxygen to reach the cornea than the older "hard" lenses, overcome this problem by providing a smooth refracting surface on the front of the eye. Furthermore, the tears collect under the lenses, filling in any irregularities.

If you are extremely nearsighted, the resolving power of your eyes may be deficient. Refractive surgery will not help this problem, even though images will be focused nearer the retina. The photoreceptors in the back of a severely nearsighted eye often are less closely packed than in the normally-sighted or mildly myopic eye. Think of the difference between high- and low-definition TV: the pixels on the screen of a low-definition TV are spread further apart so that the picture is less sharp. To use another analogy, although refractive surgery can put your "camera" more in focus, these procedures cannot make your retinal "film" better.

TREATING FARSIGHTEDNESS

You will recall that if you are farsighted, or hyperopic, light comes to an imaginary focal point behind your retina (see fig. 5). The farsighted eyeball is too short from front to back for the power of the cornea, causing a blurred image up close. (The length of your eye may be too short from front to back, or your cornea may be flatter than normal, or both.) Almost all newborn babies are farsighted; those who aren't often become markedly nearsighted as adults. Since many hyperopic patients can see distant objects well when they are young, they are called farsighted.

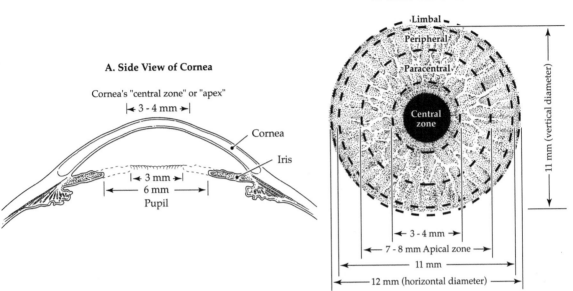

B. Front View of Cornea

A. Side View of Cornea

Cornea's "central zone" or "apex"

|← 3 - 4 mm →|

Cornea

Iris

|← 3 mm →|
|← 6 mm →|
Pupil

Limbal

Peripheral

Paracentral

Central zone

11 mm (vertical diameter)

|← 3 - 4 mm →|
|← 7 - 8 mm Apical zone →|
|← 11 mm →|
|← 12 mm (horizontal diameter) →|

The "Zones" of the Cornea

Figure 15

The dome-shaped transparent cornea.

A. *Side view* of the normal cornea.

Note: The "central zone" or apex. Only the cornea's central zone is spherical.

Note: The pupil. The size of the pupil increases in dim light. People with large pupils may have poorer night vision than patients with normal-size pupils. When the pupil opens in dim light, its diameter increases from approximately 3 mm to about 6 mm. The larger the pupil, the more cornea available to refract light, and the larger the image on the retina. Since the cornea is aspheric or unequally curved, it has multiple refractive powers across its surface along a radius from the center to the edge. At night a ghosting effect can occur around street lamps because light rays are bent at different angles across the cornea.

B. Front view of the normal cornea showing the *"zones"* of the cornea.

To reduce *nearsightedness*, the excimer laser removes corneal tissue from the *central zone* (3 to 4 mm) and *apical zone* (7 to 8 mm), creating an *optical zone* (curved tissue lens) that is about 6.5 mm in diameter. The goal is to make the curvature of the cornea flatter.

To reduce *farsightedness*, the scanning excimer laser removes corneal tissue from the *mid-apical* zone at about 7 mm, creating a carefully blended circular "valley" to change the curvature of the window of the eye. The goal is to make the curve of the *central* cornea steeper. Even though the laser is never aimed directly over the line-of-sight, the effect of surgery is over the pupil. The outer edge of the cornea is actually slightly oval shaped (rather than round as in the drawing), measuring about 12 mm horizontally and 11 mm vertically.

To correct farsightedness, a laser surgeon makes the center of the eye's window steeper by removing tissue in a carefully blended circular pattern around the mid-periphery of the cornea (see fig. 11b). Even though the laser is not aimed at the line-of-sight, the effect of treatment is directly over the pupil. After surgery, the central cornea has a steeper curve with more light-blending ability that can focus incoming light nearer the retina instead of behind it. Although both hyperopic and myopic LASIK procedures remove tissue to the same depth for the same number of diopters of refractive error, much more tissue is removed from the cornea to treat farsightedness. Refractive surgery for farsightedness can improve both near and distance vision, although you may still need glasses to read if you are over forty. (See page 113 for more details about hyperopic LASIK, or H-LASIK.)

While it is true that the farsighted eye focuses light at a theoretical point beyond the retina, hyperopia is more complex than this brief explanation implies. Without the added light-bending power of the flexible crystalline lens inside your eye, even parallel light rays reflected off distant objects "focus" behind your sensitive photoreceptors. Causing an even more blurred image, the divergent rays from close objects "come together" still further behind your retina than light from far away.

So to help you understand farsightedness on a practical level, you need to keep in mind how the two lenses of your eye—your powerful fixed corneal lens and your adjustable crystalline lens inside your eye—work together to focus light. In the youthful eye, the flexible crystalline lens can "morph" itself, becoming thicker to bring close objects into view and remaining flatter to look in the distance. Instantly changing shape, this amazing lens becomes rounder (more highly curved) for near vision to add more focusing power to your optical system. Doctors call this process "accommodation" (see insert 5, *How Your Eyes Refract Light*, page 42).

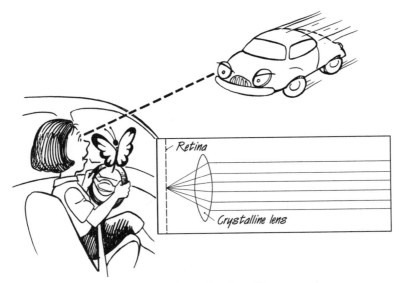

A. Looking in the distance

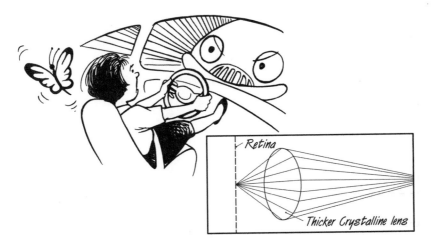

B. Looking close up

Figure 16

A. By the time light rays bouncing off a distant object reach the eye, they are nearly *parallel*, rather than focused to a point.

B. When light rays from *nearby* objects enter your eye, they are *spread* out rather than parallel. Even though the cornea bends the rays inward, it lacks the power to focus close-up objects. In order to *bend* the light rays further to focus them on the retina, the *crystalline lens inside the eye* must become *rounder* (thicker) and thus more powerful.

INSERT 5
HOW YOUR EYES REFRACT LIGHT

When light bounces off a distant car speeding directly toward you, the light rays reflected from its shiny surface are nearly *parallel*, rather than focused for clear vision. Unless your eyes bend or refract the light inward to a point on your retina, you will not see the car's rapidly approaching image (see fig. 16). Swerving to the road's shoulder, you suddenly see a huge oak tree six feet ahead. As you frantically turn back toward the road, you glance at your nearby speedometer, but the light rays bouncing off your instrument panel are *spread out*. Unless the lenses of your eyes concentrate these rays, you cannot see this close up view either. In order for you to react quickly enough to save your life, your eyes must instantaneously place clear, ever-changing images on your retinas. Any significant defects in the focusing mechanism of your eyes will decrease your visual acuity and thus your ability to take action.

It is the job of the two lenses of each eye—your *fixed* cornea and your *adjustable* crystalline lens behind your pupil—to bend these incoming rays toward one another to focus them on your retinal photoreceptors. As the car's unstoppable fender smashes through your windshield and stops two inches from your nose, your eyes—once you dare to open them—must change focus again. The closer the hot metal is to your face, the more your adjustable lens must automatically become rounder to bend the incoming light so that you can see this unpleasant sight (see fig. 16).

The crystalline lens of the farsighted eye not only must become thicker for near vision, but also for distance. In some hyperopic patients, this elastic lens is unable to compensate enough to allow clear close vision. If you need correction for farsightedness, both of your lenses working in concert lack enough focusing power to "pull" the image forward onto your retina. Put yet another way, the combined power of your corneal and crystalline lenses fails to bend light enough to focus it on your photoreceptors.

If you are farsighted, you may suffer from fatigue or headaches because of the way your eyes focus. Normally, when you look at a close object, both eyes naturally move inward toward each other. The same nerves that control the muscles that cause your eyes to converge also govern the focusing power of your crystalline lens. Your adjustable lens and your eye muscles are designed to work together to provide good single, binocular near vision. But when a farsighted person looks in the distance—as each lens adjusts to overcome hyperopia—the eyes try to turn toward the nose. Since you must look straight ahead to see far away, your brain instantly counteracts this automatic response and tells the eye muscles to move your eyes outward. Such focusing problems can cause eye strain, double vision, or both.

Some farsighted patients say, "When I'm tired, I can feel my eyes 'pulling,' but I can still see to read. If I get extremely fatigued, however, I start to see double." Our brain valiantly tries to keep us from seeing two images, but when we're exhausted, it sometimes loses the battle (see insert 6, *A Closer Look at Farsightedness*, below).

INSERT 6
A Closer Look at Farsightedness

To understand hyperopia more clearly, imagine this scene: after traveling all night, you finally stand mesmerized before one of Europe's highest mountains, the stately Mont Blanc in the French Alps. As you gaze at its awe-inspiring grandeur, you are exhausted from little sleep and jet lag. Your eyes feel strained and your head throbs with pain probably because you are farsighted.

continued

A CLOSER LOOK AT FARSIGHTEDNESS
(CONTINUED)

Unfortunately, since your eyeballs are slightly shorter than normal, your corneal lenses lack enough power to pull the mountain's image from behind each retina directly onto it. Although you can almost feel the mountain's looming presence, your crystalline lenses must spring into action to place the image on your photoreceptors. Trying to improve your focus, your brain orders your elastic crystalline lenses to become rounder to add more power to your optical system. Obeying your brain's command, the adjustable lenses of your eyes become steeper to put the majestic image on your retinas. But as your eyes try to focus in the distance, the eye muscles automatically start to pull each globe inward toward your nose. To prevent this, your brain realigns the mountain's image by telling the muscles to counteract the initial impulse of your eyes to converge. Obviously, your eyes fail to work together with ease. You may even feel a pulling sensation around each eye. Although it is early in the day, eye strain intensifies your fatigue. Ignoring the waves of weakness flowing through your body from jet lag, you glance at your travel guide. But every word is totally blurred. Although it is a struggle, your eyes can still overcome farsightedness when looking in the distance, but you can no longer focus upclose. With a deep frown, you fumble through your pockets, searching for your reading glasses. It is no wonder that your eyes burn and your head pounds with pain.

Depending on the severity of your farsightedness, you may be able to see well when you are young because your crystalline lens can still compensate for a weak corneal lens. A youngster can accommodate between +15 and +20 diopters. Consequently, many young farsighted people need no glasses because each eye's lens automatically fine-tunes the focus. As we age, however, the adjustable lens, which contributes one-third of the eye's

continued

A CLOSER LOOK AT FARSIGHTEDNESS

(CONTINUED)

focusing power, gradually loses its ability to change shape to overcome hyperopia. By age thirty, the accommodative capacity of the lens drops to +8 to +10 diopters. As farsighted people approach age forty, focusing close objects becomes more difficult. They often first notice a slight deterioration in vision in a dimly lit restaurant. With time, these individuals also lose their ability to see in the distance without corrective lenses or surgery.

Let's say, for example, that you have +3 diopters of hyperopia at age thirty. If your adjustable lens can focus up to +6 diopters, it can easily overcome +3 diopters of hyperopia at a distance and +5.5 diopters close-up. A few years pass. Having lost some of its ability to accommodate for your farsightedness, your variable lens now may only be able to focus +4 diopters. Although you still can see well in the distance at this stage of your life, you will need over 1 diopter of correction to read. More time passes. You are nearing forty. Your crystalline lens now can only focus +2 diopters, meaning that you need glasses for distance as well as near vision.

TREATING ASTIGMATISM

Many nearsighted or farsighted patients also have astigmatism, a refractive error whereby light is not focused to a single point. Vision is indistinct at every distance because the cornea—which should be dome-shaped—is "out-of-round," or shaped rather like the back of a spoon. Derived from Latin, the word astigmatism literally means "not (*a*) round (*stigmata*)." Such a cornea is more steeply curved in one direction than the other, having two "axes" that are usually perpendicular to each other. Depending on the person, 0.5 diopters or more of astigmatism starts to cause noticeably blurred vision (see insert 7, *A Closer Look at Astigmatism,* on page 46).

INSERT 7

A CLOSER LOOK AT ASTIGMATISM

If you have astigmatism, you may be curious how it causes blurred vision. Common *regular* astigmatism is much easier to understand if you think of a 3-D picture of a football lying on its side (see fig. 17). Unlike the normal cornea, which has a *central* dome, or cap, that is shaped more like a round basketball, the football-shaped astigmatic cornea bends light at different angles so that the rays fail to come together at one point on the retina. The vertical dimension of the astigmatic cornea is steeper (more curved) than the flatter horizontal dimension. Doctors use these two unequally-curved lines to describe regular astigmatism because of the way they place light on the photoreceptors. Called "meridians" (think of the earth's Greenwich prime meridian), each line follows the cornea's curved surface. They meet in the center and are 90 degrees apart. Having different curvatures, the two meridians of the astigmatic cornea have *different amounts of refractive power.* Since the steeper meridian bends light more than the flatter one, the two focal lines of light create blurred vision. For example, one meridian may place light behind the retina and one in front of it. Other combinations are possible. As astigmatism increases, vision obviously becomes more blurred.

Your doctor uses a "cylindrical lens" to correct regular astigmatism with glasses. A specially-ground cylinder-shaped lens can provide different refractive power in different meridians. Such a lens has the ability to bring the light traveling through two unequal meridians together to a point.

Briefly, regular astigmatism manifests itself in several basic ways. If you have *simple hyperopic astigmatism*, the image is blurred because light is bent so that one focal point falls on the retina and the other falls behind it. If you have *simple*

continued

A CLOSER LOOK AT ASTIGMATISM
(CONTINUED)

myopic astigmatism, the image lacks focus because one focal point falls on the retina and the other falls in front of it. If you have *compound astigmatism,* both focal points fall either in front of the retina (myopic) or behind the retina (hyperopic). If you have *mixed astigmatism,* one focal point lies behind the retina and the other one lies in front of it.

Laser surgery can smooth out the astigmatic cornea's curvature, changing the shape of the central cornea (mainly the central 6 or 7 millimeters) to look more like a symmetrical soup bowl than the back of a lopsided spoon. To correct astigmatism surgically, which is more difficult than treating nearsightedness, physicians selectively remove tissue to make the curvature of the steepest and flattest "meridians" (the corneal curves of greatest and smallest refractive power) more alike (see fig. 17). (Remember, the unevenly curved surfaces of your cornea bend light differently.) For example, if you have simple myopic astigmatism, the curvature of the meridians can be evened out by lasering tissue from the steepest meridian to make it flatter—thereby moving the light-bending effect of this forward axis back toward the retina. Less tissue would be removed from the other, flatter meridian.

Some refractive surgeons target astigmatism with a specially "masked" broad-beam laser that is driven by customized computer software. Since the surface topography of the cornea is digitized, or put in numerical form, the computer knows which areas are elevated. During a more modern surgical technique using a "flying-spot" laser, a fast, small-beam laser dances around the cornea, chipping away at the higher spots and avoiding the flatter areas. To treat the refractive error in the left eye discussed in insert 8, *Where Is*

A. Normal Cornea

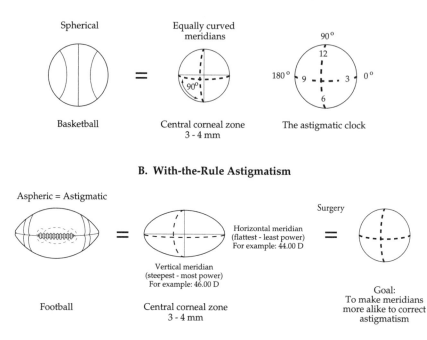

Spherical

Basketball

Equally curved meridians

90°

Central corneal zone
3 - 4 mm

The astigmatic clock

B. With-the-Rule Astigmatism

Aspheric = Astigmatic

Football

Central corneal zone
3 - 4 mm

Horizontal meridian
(flattest - least power)
For example: 44.00 D

Vertical meridian
(steepest - most power)
For example: 46.00 D

Surgery

Goal:
To make meridians
more alike to correct
astigmatism

C. Oblique Astigmatism

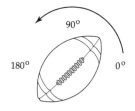

90°

180°   0°

D. Against-the-Rule Astigmatism

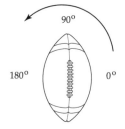

90°

180°   0°

Figure 17

A. The normally shaped spherical cornea with no astigmatism has a central dome that is shaped rather like a round basketball.

B. Regular astigmatism. The out-of-round astigmatic cornea is shaped like a football. When the "football" is lying on its side, the refractive error is known as "with-the-rule" astigmatism. The vertical dimension (curved meridian) of this astigmatic cornea has a steeper curvature and thus more refractive power than the horizontal meridian. With regular astigmatism, the two meridians are at right angles to each other.

C. Regular "oblique" astigmatism. Note how the "football," or astigmatic axis, has turned, but the meridians remain 90 degrees apart.

D. Regular "against-the-rule" astigmatism. Note how the "football" has turned so that the steeper meridian runs horizontally and the flatter one runs vertically.

Your Astigmatism? The Astigmatic Clock, the flying spot laser would track back and forth across the steepest meridian, removing enough tissue to try to eliminate 3.75 diopters of myopia. To treat the flatter meridian, the laser would "photoablate," or precisely vaporize, enough tissue to treat -3.5 diopters of nearsightedness. Soon doctors also hope to be able to treat "irregular astigmatism," a fine wrinkling of the cornea, by flattening the hills and leaving the valleys alone. Once the eye's window is thus recontoured, rays of sunshine can come to a clear point on the retina.

INSERT 8
WHERE IS YOUR ASTIGMATISM?
THE ASTIGMATIC CLOCK

To write an eyeglasses prescription for astigmatism, your doctor must describe the location (the axis) of the power needed to achieve the desired light-bending effect in terms of either the flattest or steepest meridian. Physicians use an "astigmatic optical clock" to describe the orientation of the axis of astigmatism (see fig. 17). The location of each meridian is expressed in degrees on this circular clock. Notice that 0 degrees is at the three o'clock position. Moving counterclockwise, 90 degrees is at the twelve noon location, and 180 degrees is at nine o'clock.

What does your doctor mean when she says that you have "with-the-rule," "oblique," or "against-the rule" astigmatism? In with-the-rule astigmatism, the steeper vertical meridian (the shorter dimension of the football) runs from the twelve o'clock position to the six o'clock position on the astigmatic clock. As just noted, this meridian has the most light-bending power and thus the most plus, or refractive, power. The flattest horizontal meridian (the longer dimension of the football), which runs from three o'clock to nine o'clock, has the least refractive

continued

Where Is Your Astigmatism?
The Astigmatic Clock (continued)

power and is 90 degrees from the vertical meridian (see fig. 17). Determining the position of the steepest and flattest meridians of the cornea, the entire axis can be turned like the hands of a clock, although the lines remain perpendicular with regular astigmatism (see fig. 17). At a certain rotation point, common, with-the-rule astigmatism becomes oblique astigmatism. For example, one position of the axis of oblique astigmatism might be stated as at 135 degrees or at 45 degrees.

In against-the-rule astigmatism, the "football" turns so that the steeper meridian runs horizontally and the flatter one runs vertically (see fig. 17).

Finally, there is yet another kind of astigmatism called "irregular" astigmatism in which the surface is not smooth, and the major and minor meridians are not perpendicular to each other. Often caused by a fine wrinkling of the corneal surface, irregular astigmatism can only be corrected with rigid contact lenses—not with glasses or soft contacts. Surgeons have attempted to diminish irregular astigmatism with some of the newer special lasers with unpredictable results. The advent of the new custom "wavefront" LASIK may help some of these patients.

The difference between the two lines on the astigmatic "cross" is the amount of astigmatism of the cornea. For example, if the vertical meridian of your cornea (the steepest one) has 46 diopters of focusing power and the horizontal has 44 diopters of converging power, the difference between the two, which is 2 diopters, is the amount of your corneal astigmatism in that eye. For the technically-minded, the "keratometry" reading of this eye could be written:

44.00 @ 180 degrees / 46.00 @ 90 degrees

There are other causes of astigmatism besides irregularities on the front (anterior) surface of your cornea. The back (posterior) of your cornea also can be malformed (see fig. 4). Furthermore, since your eye is a two-lens system, problems with the front and back curvature of your crystalline lens *inside* your eye can cause astigmatism. In fact, any misalignment of the internal components of your eye can blur images placed on your retina. A few people have astigmatism because of a disparity between their line-of-sight (the visual axis which goes from what they are looking at to the light-sensing photoreceptors on the retinal fovea) and their optic axis (the way the light strikes the retina) (see fig. 6). Densely packed with receptors, the fovea—a tiny depression in the retina—is the area of clearest vision. In these patients, the rays of light fail to strike the fovea correctly. Laser surgery is unable to treat these problems.

Currently, refractive surgeons can only correct the part of your astigmatic error caused by irregularities in the curvature of the *front* surface of your cornea. Consequently, the more disparity between treatable surface corneal astigmatism and total astigmatism, the less predictable the surgical result. To even out the cornea's front surface, the laser can be programmed to make the cornea more bowl-shaped. Unfortunately, some patients have noticeable astigmatism caused by problems *inside* their eyes. These patients will still have residual astigmatism after surgery, even if the front of the cornea is treated. In fact, many eyes that manifest no refractive astigmatism (as measured during an eye exam) actually have astigmatic defects inside the eye, but they are counterbalanced by astigmatism on the surface of the cornea. This is one instance in which two wrongs do make a right, because the error in one lens offsets that in the other to provide clear focus.

MANAGING AGE-RELATED PRESBYOPIA:
A KEY TO YOUR FUTURE VISION

Refractive surgery to reduce focusing errors goes beyond helping nearsighted, farsighted, and astigmatic people become less dependent on corrective lenses. If you have presbyopia (caused by a natural loss of flexibility of the lens inside each eye), recently developed LASIK surgical techniques can diminish this refractive error.

Remember when your mom and dad started wearing glasses to read. Without them, they probably held the newspaper at arm's length to see properly. Eventually their arms became too short. Your parents had age-related presbyopia ("old eyes"). With the passing years, all of us gradually lose our ability to focus close up. For this reason, if you are considering surgery, an in-depth knowledge of this refractive error is absolutely key to understanding your future vision. Otherwise, you may not comprehend why surgeons often suggest leaving patients a little nearsighted (undercorrected) in one eye, especially if they are approaching forty.

So why would an eye doctor—who wants to give you the best-possible vision—suggest surgically undercorrecting your vision in one eye? This is an important question that physicians spend almost half their time explaining to patients. Let's say, for example, that you are thirty-six and nearsighted, and LASIK focuses both of your eyes to 20/20 in the distance. For the first few years after your surgery, you probably will be thrilled with your vision. But by age forty you may begin to have problems seeing close up. Your doctor knows that this event is inevitable—it is associated with the aging process.

To help you understand why this happens, let's focus once again on how your youthful, flexible crystalline lens inside your eye enables you to see up close. As it does with farsightedness, this adjustable lens plays a central role in presbyopia. It is important, however, not to confuse the two focusing errors. Remember how both of the lenses of your eye work together to enable you to see a nearby object. If you hold this page close to your eyes, lamplight bounces off the words and spreads apart rapidly. In order for you to read, the optical system of each eye must gather these divergent light rays and focus them on your retina. Your eye only has the short length of an eyeball to do this. As you now know, after the incoming shafts of light are bent by your fixed cornea, they are further refracted by your adjustable crystalline lens. To help you focus up close, the youthful crystalline lens, which is a variable focusing mechanism, changes shape, becoming more spherical. The more round or curved this lens becomes, the more ability it has to converge incoming light rays, bringing them to a point quickly.

When you are young, your crystalline lens can accommodate, or change focus, to see close. In your late thirties, however, you become "pre-presbyopic," meaning that you will soon need reading glasses. Interestingly enough, even though you begin to lose the ability to accommodate as early as in your twenties, you probably won't notice until you approach forty (or older) because your crystalline lens has reserve focusing power.

But around forty, farsighted and normally sighted persons become aware that they can no longer see close well. Even nearsighted people will have this problem *when they wear glasses for distance.* Less flexible and larger, the crystalline lens no longer provides enough added light-blending power for reading. To see near objects well, some mildly nearsighted older people simply remove their glasses. If LASIK surgery corrects both eyes for the distance, these folks will have to wear glasses to read. As the degree of myopia increases, it becomes impractical to take off one's glasses because the book must be held too close to the face for comfort.

Patients with presbyopia usually wear magnifiers, bifocals, trifocals, or graduated lenses in their glasses. Other patients wear reading glasses over contact lenses or else bifocal contacts. Lenses that correct both presbyopia and nearsightedness add plus power (to aid near vision) to glasses or contacts along with the distance prescription.

If you have poor near vision caused by age-related presbyopia, special laser treatments might help you see better up close. In other words, depending on your particular correction, if you are about forty years old, LASIK may improve your functional vision so that you can read a newspaper or see your computer screen without glasses, although you may still need magnifiers for fine print. "Monovision," whereby one eye is focused for the distance and the other one is left slightly undercorrected, or nearsighted, for close work, may allow you to see better both near and far without correction.

Monovision for Age-related Presbyopia

Achieving Monovision with Contacts Lenses

If you need correction to read, monovision—which is a *compromise* solution to age-related presbyopia—might help you manage this refractive error. You may be able to improve your near vision by wearing a contact lens in your non-dominant eye that leaves your myopia a little undercorrected. By focusing one eye for the distance and the other one for near, you should be able to see both far away and up close—when you use *both* eyes. The goal is to allow you to become less dependent on bifocal contact lenses or reading glasses. Even if you have presbyopia, if you are also nearsighted, you probably can still focus near objects *when you remove your glasses*. In a way, monovision achieves a similar effect in the undercorrected eye.

Everyone has a dominant and a non-dominant eye. Your dominant eye can be corrected for the distance. Normally, your dominant eye leads the way, telling your eyes where to point and how to focus at any distance. With monovision, however, most people tend to be most comfortable using the dominant eye for the demands of distance vision, such as driving, and the non-dominant one for close-up tasks, such as reading. Only when the non-dominant eye has an optical advantage in seeing up close does it lead the way for near vision. If you have perfect 20/20 distance vision with both eyes, but need magnifying glasses, you can wear a contact lens in your non-dominant eye to make you a little nearsighted so that you can see up close. Since you use both eyes together, you shouldn't give up much noticeable distance vision by leaving one eye slightly undercorrected by 0.5 to 1.5 diopters. Monovision may improve your range of vision *with both eyes open.*

Monovision works well for about half of presbyopic patients. If the difference in refraction between the two eyes is minimal, the brain will often sort out the best possible vision within a few weeks. A small focusing dissimilarity is imperceptible, and the two eyes together see better than either one individually. A large variation, however, casts a shadow over the visual field. Most motivated people who understand the benefits of monovision can tolerate up to a 2-diopter difference between their two eyes, which often occurs naturally. Some patients, however, especially those who work at a desk all day, find even a slight imbalance unacceptable. Some people also are bothered by the decrease in depth perception that can occur with monovision.

Your eye doctor can demonstrate monovision by letting you try contact lenses that slightly undercorrect nearsightedness in your non-dominant eye. For many patients, monovision is an excellent solution to presbyopia. Some people say: "This is wonderful! I can glance from the theater stage to my program without searching for reading glasses." Others, however might, say: "This drives me crazy. I like to play softball and tennis. I want *both* of my eyes focused for the distance. I will wear reading glasses for close work."

Achieving Monovision through Refractive Surgery

It is often possible to achieve the effects of monovision with refractive surgery. If you are a nearsighted patient with age-related presbyopia and need extra correction for reading, your eye doctor can surgically treat your *non-dominant* eye first, leaving it a *little nearsighted* for close work. He can target your visual acuity in your *dominant* eye for the distance. After the operation, you should ideally be able to see your television and your calculator without bifocals—although you may still require magnifiers for fine print. If you don't like surgically-induced monovision, you probably will still have the option of having a second LASIK procedure later to refocus your undercorrected eye for the distance.

Bob, a forty-three-year-old banker, had only -1 diopter of myopia in each eye. He asked for LASIK on his eyes to focus *both* of them for the distance. Before his LASIK procedure he could read the 20/40 line of the eye chart. Like many mildly nearsighted, middle-aged persons he just took his glasses off to read. Hence, we suggested that he have *only* one eye—his dominant one—treated for the distance. He could use his other eye for some close work, although he might need magnifiers for fine print—especially as he ages. Even though we thoroughly explained the benefits of monovision to Bob, noting the other eye could be treated later, we had a difficult time convincing him to leave one eye uncorrected. He was so determined to have both eyes surgically focused for the distance that he absolutely insisted on paying for two operations. But a few weeks after I operated on Bob's dominant eye, he said, "You're absolutely right. I don't need more surgery. Monovision works pretty well for me." We returned his second check. It is always important to be conservative when deciding to perform refractive surgery—but especially in the lower ranges of myopia.

The benefits of monovision are further illustrated by the unusual case of a well-known refractive surgeon from Australia. At age forty-five he had perfect 20/20 distance vision in both eyes, but he needed glasses to read. When I visited him in Australia, the ophthalmologist asked me to perform *hyperopic* LASIK for farsightedness on his non-dominant eye to make it a little nearsighted for close work.

He said, "I tried monovision for about one month by wearing a contact lens in my non-dominant eye to make me slightly myopic. I enjoyed seeing the gas gauge of my car and my map without searching for my reading glasses. I only wore magnifiers to read fine print such as the letters on a medicine bottle. I've decided to sacrifice a little of my 'perfect' distance vision in one eye so that I can see better up close."

The eye doctor actually wanted to *decrease* his visual acuity in his non-dominant eye from perfect distance vision (plano) to -1.5 diopters. After refractive surgery, the ophthalmologist was elated. He could see clearly far away and close up—using *both* eyes.

This surgeon had an excellent understanding of the advantages and limitations of refractive surgery and had simulated the desired LASIK results with a trial contact lens. Even for an eye doctor, a verbal description of vision is a poor substitute for living it. When we try to explain what monovision is like, patients have difficulty understanding it. Although we targeted the ophthalmologist's surgical change at -1.5 diopters, we had a quarter to three-quarter diopter leeway in the treatment of his near vision. The surgical refraction of near vision doesn't have to be as precise as that for distance vision. Since patients can comfortably vary how far they hold a book from their eyes by a few inches, acceptable near vision is possible even if the healing process changes the surgical outcome slightly.

Monovision may also help an extremely nearsighted person who is beginning to become presbyopic. Jerry, a forty-one-year-old realtor, had -11 diopters of myopia. He was having difficulty reading the phone book with his contact lenses. They corrected him for distance only. Saying that he "hated having heavy hunks of plastic hanging on his nose," Jerry angrily described his eyesight with glasses as "tunnel vision." With no corrective lenses, he held the newspaper about two inches from his eyes. Reading like this gave him a severe headache. Jerry wanted LASIK to correct his myopia.

After LASIK, his residual refractive error was mild, improving to -1.75 diopters in his dominant eye and -1.5 diopters in his non-dominant one. Three months after his operation, he asked for further surgery on his dominant eye because he wished to see better in the distance. After Jerry's enhancement procedure, he was +0.25 diopters in his dominant eye, meaning that he was a *tiny* bit farsighted. Two weeks after surgery, Jerry was able to read the 20/15 line on the eye chart with this eye. He had *better* than 20/20 or normal visual acuity in the distance. Needless to say, Jerry was ecstatic!

But one month after his enhancement operation, Jerry was back, demanding that his visual acuity in his non-dominant eye be refined. In other words, he wanted it focused for the distance also. However, since he is in his early forties, he will gradually lose his ability to focus up close. In a few years, if we correct both of his eyes for the distance, Jerry probably will need magnifying glasses not only to read fine print but also to see anything on his desk. Once Jerry is about fifty, every object within six feet may become a little blurred. Anything beyond six feet should be fairly clear. This means that Jerry will have to wear glasses not only to read a menu but also to see across a dinner table. If you have ever worn glasses or contacts that were a little too strong, you know how irritating it is to try to talk with a friend when you are unable to see her face.

We discouraged Jerry from having further surgery on his non-dominant eye. As he ages, he can use it to focus close objects. We had a difficult time, however, convincing him to leave this eye slightly undercorrected, or myopic. Like most people, Jerry was in denial that he eventually would no longer see clearly up close. All of us have trouble understanding presbyopia before our eyes naturally lose the ability to focus near objects. Nearsighted young patients— who have never experienced poor near vision—single-mindedly judge their surgical results by their visual acuity in the distance. They think that excellent *distance* vision is the answer to all their eyesight problems. Few of us realize how important near vision is until it is no longer in focus. Doctors must help patients understand that monovision can give them more functional vision as they grow older. Before surgery, almost everyone has a slightly different refractive error in each eye just as one arm is stronger than the other. Leaving the non-dominant eye slightly myopic, or undercorrected, should have a negligible effect on Jerry's distance vision, but he will have much better near vision with both eyes open.

If only we could prevent presbyopia. Refractive surgery can help patients such as Jerry see better over a greater range of vision, but no surgery can stop the natural progression of the deterioration of the crystalline lens. LASIK might make us feel younger, but it cannot subtract years from the age of our eyes.

IMPROVING DEPTH-OF-FIELD

Laser eye surgery also helps presbyopia by improving each individual eye's depth-of-field, or the range of focusing ability. In optics, the range of clear vision through a single lens (a single power) is called the depth-of-field of that lens. Think how a focused camera has a range within which you can move backward or forward from the subject a few feet and still create a sharp picture. Even before surgery, the profile of your untouched cornea isn't totally round all the way out to the edge (see fig. 15a). Doctors say that the normal cornea is "aspheric"—not spherical, or perfectly round. This innate asphericity in the curvature of your eye's most powerful lens helps increase depth-of-field. Enhancing nature's design of your eyes in some respects, the precise excimer laser slightly flattens your cornea's curvature, making it even less spherical. Although this effect may slightly alter night vision, such increased asphericity of your cornea helps improve close vision.

THE ART OF REFRACTIVE SURGERY

Performing expert vision correction surgery entails much more than understanding the complicated optics of your eye, the minute dimensions of your astonishing corneal lens, and the esoteric dynamics of the computer-controlled excimer laser. The art of being your doctor requires a number of abilities: 1) knowing if a particular procedure is right for you; 2) discerning your visual goals in order to adapt your eyesight to your lifestyle; 3) helping you examine your expectations about refractive surgery to see if they are realistic; 4) understanding how your age might affect your results; 5) clearly explaining what happens to your eyes during an operation; and 6) carefully presenting all the risks as well as the rewards of a particular procedure. As healthy human beings, we often plan for the best outcome and ignore the possibility that problems can occur. We may only hear what we want to hear. Your doctor must make you aware that—even though refractive surgery can be tremendously rewarding—as with any operation, side effects and rare complications are possible.

Refractive surgeons can eliminate or reduce your dependence on glasses or contacts, but they can never promise that you will be totally free of corrective lenses after surgery. Even though most patients achieve dramatically improved eyesight after LASIK, the results are *not* always perfect for everyone. In fact, no operation performed on the human body will ever be perfect. Although vision correcting surgery has become a highly refined, technologically advanced science, it is still *surgery*. It is definitely not for everyone, nor is it a panacea for all vision problems. If your eyes were molded of plastic in a standardized pre-cast form, your doctor's task would be much easier. But made of continuously changing, living tissue, your eyes are totally unique to you. You heal slightly differently than anyone else in the world. Hence, your distinctive visual problems and healing response will affect your surgical recovery and your future eyesight. Since your eyes are like no others, even the most skilled refractive surgeon using the latest equipment can *never* guarantee anything. Even in the best hands, rare complications can occur during and after *any* operation, including eye surgery, and the results of those complications can be permanent.

When pursuing the quest for better vision, a key consideration is locating a qualified ophthalmologist. As a prospective patient, how can you evaluate the doctor's training, equipment, and expertise? The more knowledgeable you are about each refractive procedure, the better you will be able to choose your surgeon. Hence, our goal is to provide you with a good understanding of refractive surgery so that you can work *with* your physician to decide if you are a good candidate to achieve the effect you desire. Together, you and your eye doctor can pick the correct procedure for you.

As a highly informed patient, you should know exactly what happens before, during, and after refractive surgery. In fact, you probably want to know exactly how it works. You may even wish to grasp some of the crucial technical issues covered later. Whatever your vision problem, your main concern about these operations probably is their safety. In addition, you might be asking: What are the results for my degree of refractive error? Are there any possible short- and long-term post-operative side effects following these procedures? Throughout the following chapters, we will address all of these concerns, covering in detail each individual type of refractive surgery including LASIK, PRK, and RK.

As we enter the third millennium, more and more new procedures to refine the human body are being developed. In the past, people could have their teeth and noses straightened and their wrinkles and excess fat removed. Nowadays, modern refractive surgery—which improves the way the eyes work rather than how they look—offers better vision for nearsighted, farsighted, astigmatic, and even presbyopic patients. With the advent of the new LASIK procedure, many people will indeed be able to see more clearly without their glasses and contact lenses—a goal only dreamed of by past generations.

CHAPTER TWO

LASIK: THE STATE-OF-THE-ART EXCIMER LASER PROCEDURE

The maxim that: "Success depends upon attention to details," is particularly true for refractive surgery because in it, the distance that separates success from unwanted complications or mediocre results is only a small fraction of a millimeter.

—Jose Barraquer, M.D.
a pioneer in refractive surgery

Imagine that you can no longer wear your contact lenses—not gas permeable ones, not soft contacts, not even the disposable kind. At age forty-three, my eyes had become so dry that, after only two hours, even the thinnest, most hydrophilic contacts with a high-water content stuck to my corneas. I had Vaseline vision—and the jar was turning gray.

The edges of my glasses were so thick that I peered at the world through a dark, blurry tunnel. Unable to look through those Coke-bottle bottoms, I would often rip them off in anger. But without glasses, I had to hold a book two inches from my nose, and even then I couldn't focus on the words. It hurt my brain to look at the distorted page.

I was a parent, an only child of chronically ill parents, a car-pool mom, a business executive, a writer, and a swimmer. When I was forced to look through these pinhole spectacles, I couldn't drive, I couldn't see my computer, I couldn't write, and I couldn't swim. I couldn't even think clearly.

It's difficult to keep up the pace when you cannot see the track. At night, I almost stumbled down stairs and started to walk into glass windows. Even though I continually explained that I was unable to see well, people treated me as if I were a little out of it. I told myself over and over that my mind was keen and nimble and that my body was strong and agile. But when my friends remembered the address of a restaurant, I couldn't. I never saw the letters on the street sign.

Vacations weren't fun anymore. At the airport, my spouse asked me to jump out of the car and check in with the airline while he parked. A simple task, right? But I was filled with uncertainty.

I'll feel like a moron if I can't even do this, I said to myself.

I fumbled around for the car door handle. Finally, I felt it, opened the door, and stepped right in the muddy water by the curb. The other people in the car didn't seem to be smiling in sympathy. Why can't they remember that I can't see? I've told them a dozen times. Wiping the mud from my shoes with my thumb, I looked around for the airport entrance. Where the heck is it? I thought to myself, wishing my dry, itchy contacts weren't dehydrated. I was furious with my mate for asking me to do this.

At last, I spotted the automatic doors, but somehow I managed to try to walk in the exit. When the door failed to open, I knew instantly what I'd done. My face flushed with embarrassment, I looked back toward the car. Thank heavens! It was gone.

Sitting in the airport terminal, my husband read a newspaper article about "photorefractive keratectomy," or PRK, the original laser-based eye surgery to correct nearsightedness. The story says that during this procedure, a specially trained ophthalmologist attempts to correct refractive errors such as nearsightedness. After removing the thin, gel-like outer layer of the cornea, the surgeon uses the excimer laser to flatten the corneal surface, which, as I knew, is the powerful light-refracting window of the eye that covers the colored iris and dark pupil. Hoping that PRK might improve my vision, I immediately made an appointment with my regular eye doctor.

"PRK has helped many people, but I don't think that it is the right refractive surgery for you, Karen," said my eye doctor. "Although 90 percent of patients with mild and moderate nearsightedness less than -6 diopters eventually achieve 20/40 or better vision on the eye chart without glasses, your visual outcome following PRK would be much less predictable because you have severe myopia. You also are too nearsighted for RK, or "radial keratotomy." (As mentioned earlier and covered in detail in chapter 10, during RK, surgeons treat nearsight-edness using microscopic spoke-like incisions made free-hand in the outer cornea with a guarded, diamond-tipped blade.)

"Since you are severely myopic," continued my doctor, "even though your uncorrected vision should improve after PRK, your refraction with contacts or glasses could get worse. In other words, your glasses probably would be thinner, but you could lose lines of best-corrected visual acuity (BCVA) on the eye chart.

"To some extent, PRK results depend on each individual patient's wound-healing response. A fog-like haze can cloud the cornea imme-diately following this procedure. In mildly to moderately nearsighted people, this haze usually is subclinical. This means that even though doctors can see corneal clouding with a slit-lamp microscope, the patient doesn't notice the haze. In patients with low myopia, this problem generally disappears after a while. But in your case, the cornea might become noticeably clouded for some time. In addition, severely nearsighted patients with greater than -8 or -9 diopters of correction sometimes regress a little. Furthermore, since the outer corneal layer is removed during PRK, this procedure usually hurts for two or three days because, after the cornea is treated with the laser, the eye is left open and exposed to the air to heal.

"I know that you are having a very difficult time, Karen. But I think that you should wait awhile. Refractive surgery technology is improving. In a couple of years, we should be able to help you."

Two more years passed. At this point, I was desperate. Since I am a medical writer used to doing research, I searched the ophthalmology journals for the latest information on refractive laser eye surgery. I learned that an amazing state-of-the-art operation called LASIK, an acronym for "laser in situ keratomileusis," might be the answer to my vision problems (see figs. 10 and 18). Sometimes called "lamellar" (as within the layers of the cornea) refractive surgery by doctors, this operation originally was nicknamed "flap and zap" surgery, but few people call it that today. After partially cutting an attached protective flap of living tissue from the outer cornea, surgeons treat refractive errors by resculpting, or "zapping," the newly exposed inner cornea with the excimer laser.

One medical article says that, in highly skilled hands, this procedure generally has excellent results for mild and moderate myopia. Severely nearsighted patients also show great improvement. Another journal article indicates that visual acuity after surgery is fairly predictable and stable.

I also learned that LASIK patients have minimal operative and post-operative pain, although their eyes may feel a little scratchy and gritty for a day or so. They usually experience rapid initial visual recovery and get their final results quickly. People with low myopia often go back to work the day after surgery, although extremely-nearsighted patients may need more time to recover. Most achieve their final outcome in three months.

I needed advice on how to choose a LASIK surgeon—a corneal specialist who is expert in operating on the inner layers of the window of the eye. So I interviewed well-known eye doctors at several major universities across the country. One ophthalmologist told me that LASIK generally has fewer overall complications than other refractive operations mainly because this procedure has fewer problems related to healing. She said, however, that even though LASIK surgery is brief and looks deceptively simple to perform, in fact, the surgical technique is difficult to master. Complications occur rarely during the actual surgery, but they can be severe. Not all of them can be treated successfully. She added that the doctor's ability to avoid and manage such intra-operative complications is highly dependent on his experience.

A friend told me of a twenty-year-old girl in Colorado who was about to have a corneal transplant because one of her eyes had been damaged by a "well-meaning," but inexperienced, doctor. She was his third LASIK patient.

Keeping this story in mind, I compiled a list of the leading refractive surgeons in the U.S. and Canada by reading ophthalmology journals. With the help of a good friend, who is a physician, I finally found my surgeon. My friend recommended Stephen G. Slade, M.D., in Houston, Texas, the first ophthalmologist to perform the LASIK procedure as it is currently practiced. Dr. Slade taught the LASIK surgical technique to doctors throughout the United States. Most surgeons doing LASIK have taken the course he taught. I decided to have a preliminary consultation with him.

Dr. Slade studied the results of my eye exam, discussed my surgical goals, and then said I was a good candidate for LASIK. His partner, Dr. Baker, studied my cornea with a high-tech test called "computerized corneal topography." The computer drew a color printout of the surface of my cornea. This "corneal map" showed the steepness of the window of my eye and the exact location of my astigmatism (see fig. 19). My severe nearsightedness was caused by an elongated eyeball rather than an abnormally steep cornea. In fact, the tests showed that my cornea was flatter than normal. This meant that the microsurgical tolerances—which are measured in microns (a micron equals one millionth of a meter)—were even smaller than usual.

A Step-by-Step Look at LASIK Surgery

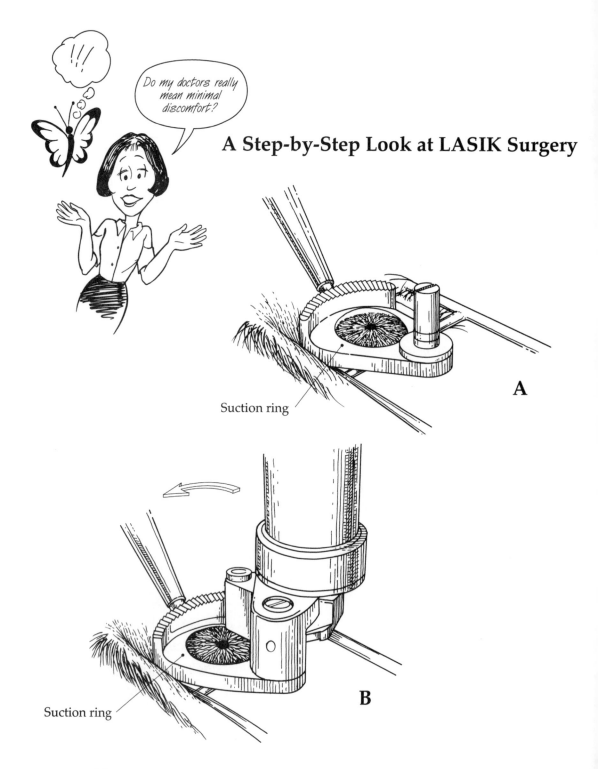

Suction ring

A

Suction ring

B

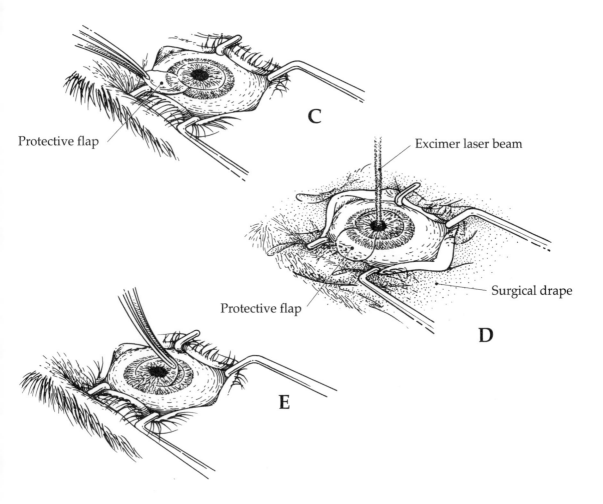

Protective flap

Excimer laser beam

Protective flap

Surgical drape

Figure 18

LASIK or "*laser in* situ *k*eratomileusis." The latest excimer laser-based refractive surgery to reduce nearsightedness and farsightedness. Working under a "hinged" or attached flap of corneal tissue, the microsurgeon uses a computer-controlled laser to change the curvature of the cornea to improve vision. After the laser treatment, the doctor gently puts the protective flap back in place on the cornea.

Note: The eyelids and eyelashes are draped before surgery, which is not shown in this line drawing.

A. The surgeon places the suction ring on the eye.

B. The keratectomy. The automated microkeratome is creating the protective flap from the cornea.

C. The doctor lifts the flap so that the excimer laser can sculpt the inner cornea.

D. The laser treatment.

E. The surgeon carefully places the protective flap back on the cornea.

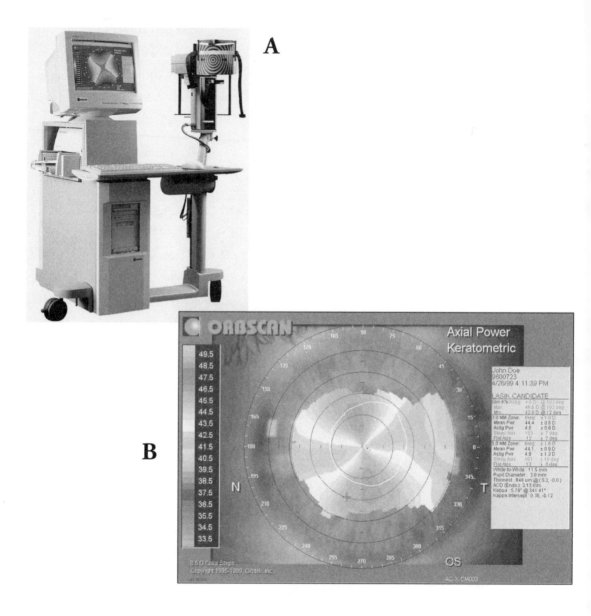

Figure 19

A. Corneal topographic equipment used to study the surface and curvature of the human cornea.

B. Mapping the window of the eye with "corneal topography." The computer generates color-coded maps that show the curvature and "hills and valleys" of the cornea. The "before and after" and "difference" maps show the effect of laser refractive surgery on the cornea.

Note: the "bow tie" pattern of the astigmatism.

I asked Dr. Slade, "What are the chances that you can correct me to 20/40 or better after surgery?"

He replied, "As you know, Karen, you unfortunately have a large refractive error of -10 diopters of myopia. You also have mild astigmatism. You need reading glasses because you have age-related presbyopia. Although I would hope for at least 20/40 or better distance vision in your dominant eye, I cannot promise you that we will get there. Our results usually are predictable and excellent. Almost 95 percent of my mildly and moderately nearsighted LASIK patients achieve 20/40 or better and 70 percent gain normal 20/20 or better vision. Nevertheless, this surgery is not perfect. [Nowadays, statistics have improved. Using the newest, fast flying-spot laser, 99.7 percent of mildly and moderately nearsighted patients can read the 20/40 line or better on the eye chart without corrective lenses, and 87.3 percent achieve normal 20/20 vision or better.] But since you are severely nearsighted, I may only get you to 20/100 or even 20/200. After surgery, you may still have to wear glasses, but they should be much thinner. We may have to do an enhancement or refinement operation. Although there is no additional surgeon's fee and only a small setup charge for repeat surgery, there are some additional risks."

"Can you correct my presbyopia?" I asked.

"You might wish to consider monovision. In other words, I could try to undercorrect your non-dominant eye a little bit so that you could read better, and I would try to focus the other one for the distance."

"What about my astigmatism?"

"We have special computer programs to improve your astigmatism, but I may not eliminate all of it," answered Dr. Slade. "Just treating your nearsightedness also may make your astigmatism a little better."

"Since I am so nearsighted, do you think that I should wait another year?" I asked. "In other words, will your results improve a lot in a year or two?"

"Our results with LASIK are improving incrementally as the computer software and the lasers get better. I don't foresee dramatic improvements in this operation in the next few years. Deciding when to have a high-tech procedure such as LASIK is a little like deciding when to buy a personal computer. No matter what is current right now, if you wait awhile, there will be something better. The question is: Do you want to do without a computer for several years? Maybe. Maybe not. Obviously, you don't want to buy a 166 MHz PC the day before the 450 MHz Pentiums are released. This is the kind of individual decision that only you can make. The good thing about LASIK is that you can have enhancements later, although the risk-to-benefit ratio increases with any repeat procedure. Having LASIK now generally won't keep you from having most other new treatments later."

"Is this surgery safe?" I asked, thinking to myself that probably even contact lenses or glasses aren't totally safe.

"From all that we currently know, this operation—when performed by a competent LASIK surgeon—is relatively safe," answered Dr. Slade. "But this is an elective procedure. As with any surgery, there are absolutely no guarantees. And unfortunately there are risks—we try to keep them to a minimum—but they are always there. For example, although infection is extremely rare, if it occurs— and we can't cure it—you could permanently lose all or part of your vision, even your entire eye. If you have such a serious complication, it won't matter that the overall LASIK infection rate is less than one in ten thousand with a skilled surgeon. If the patient has pain or senses that something is wrong, it is her responsibility to call the doctor immediately. Fortunately, we can cure most infections—if we treat them in time."

"What is the second worst possible outcome?" I asked.

"A loss of best-corrected visual acuity (BCVA) with contact lenses or glasses of greater than two lines on the eye chart," answered Dr. Slade (see fig. 9). "The risk of reduced vision with glasses is probably

less than one percent for all patients, but it increases for extremely nearsighted and farsighted people. None of the LASIK patients in the last two studies in my practice have lost more than two lines on the eye chart of best-corrected visual acuity. Many patients gain a line over a six-month period. The good news is that some patients actually see better with their glasses or contacts following refractive surgery, but not all of them."

"How safe is LASIK over the long term?"

"Doctors have been splitting the human cornea into layers, removing tissue, and putting the layers back in place for more than fifty years. We believe that LASIK is relatively safe. But nothing in medicine is totally safe. Is the cornea going to deteriorate because you have LASIK? No. After your cornea heals, does LASIK make your eye more prone to infections? No. But that doesn't mean that you might not someday get an eye infection from some totally unrelated cause."

I said, "Could my surgical results start out good, but regress over time? In other words, will my results be permanent?"

"So far, LASIK results in my practice have been reasonably stable, although some patients with severe myopia greater than -8 or -9 diopters have experienced moderate regression. This hasn't been much of a problem with mild and moderate myopia. I can perform exactly the same surgery on two women with similar vision of the same age and have different results," Dr. Slade added. "People are not pieces of plastic—the healing response varies from person to person. With LASIK, however, the final results are less affected by these individual differences than with the other refractive operations."

"I have heard that fitting contact lenses after RK is tricky," I said. "Is this true with LASIK? Since my eyes are dry, my contacts become sticky after about two hours, but I can still see better with them than with my glasses. Will I be able to wear contacts following LASIK, if I need them?"

"If your eyes are dry before surgery, they will be dry afterward, and your recovery may be a little slower than most other patients. If *you still need contact lenses after LASIK—and they were uncomfortable before surgery—you will continue to have problems with them after your operation. In other words, patients who successfully wear contacts before the procedure are able to wear them afterward and vice versa. It is much easier to fit contacts after LASIK than after RK."*

After thinking about my consultation with my doctor for a couple of weeks, I called his office and asked to talk with four of his LASIK patients. None thought that the outpatient procedure was painful, although two of them took a painkiller when they got home. One young man whose uncorrected vision improved from 20/400 to 20/30 said that he was thrilled with his results. Another moderately near-sighted man had a surgical enhancement and now sees 20/30 with both eyes without glasses. A female patient with severe myopia had hazy daytime vision and poor visual acuity at night for about six weeks. Nine months after surgery, she was seeing 20/50 uncorrected and 20/20 with soft contacts or glasses. Oddly enough, the person with the best final outcome was the least happy. Although her vision improved from about 20/500 to 20/20 without correction, she missed the super sharp 20/15 eyesight she had with gas-permeable contact lenses—but not enough to wear them.

I decided to proceed with the operation because I thought that, even if I still had to wear glasses after surgery, the chances are excellent that they would be much thinner and that I would be able to see better.

Karen

LASIK: THE SURGICAL PROCEDURE

In the 1980s, the advent of the computer software-driven excimer laser enabled specially trained eye surgeons to refocus their patients' eyes with PRK. The main variables were—and still are—the patient's wound-healing response and the surgeon's skill and understanding of the laser. Nowadays, by combining the refractive lamellar surgical techniques first pioneered over fifty years ago by Jose Barraquer, M.D., of Bogota, Colombia, with the precision of the excimer laser, corneal surgeons are able to improve vision with LASIK. Performed on the surgically exposed inner cornea, this leading-edge procedure is the culmination of the efforts of dedicated scientists from around the world, including eye doctors, physicists, engineers, computer scientists, and investors.

As you now know, LASIK is providing excellent results for many mildly and moderately nearsighted people. And for severely nearsighted persons such as Karen who cannot wear contact lenses, this procedure offers a new-found hope. Before this delicate operation became available, these patients had to go through life wearing debilitating, thick-edged glasses. LASIK can also help farsighted (hyperopic) patients see better. In fact, people with this refractive error often are our happiest LASIK patients. Before surgery, these individuals sometimes lack functional vision—especially as they age. They have difficulty performing the simple daily tasks that you and I take for granted. Some are unable to see the smile on their best friend's face at dinner or the food on their plate.

How is this breakthrough technology, which is changing people's vision and thus their lives, possible? Exactly what happens during the exquisitely complicated LASIK procedure? How is a "hinged" flap of living tissue cut from the surface of the credit-card-thick cornea using an automated "microkeratome?" A microkeratome is an electromechanically controlled surgical instrument that looks rather like a miniature carpenter's plane with a finely honed blade locked in its metal jaws (see fig. 20). How does the computer-controlled excimer laser—which can cut notches in a human hair—reshape the inner cornea to produce better vision? (See fig. 21). What does the doctor see as he looks through the operating microscope as the invisible scanning laser beam removes tissue from the eye at the submicron level? How does the corneal flap protect the newly lasered inner cornea during the post-surgical healing process?

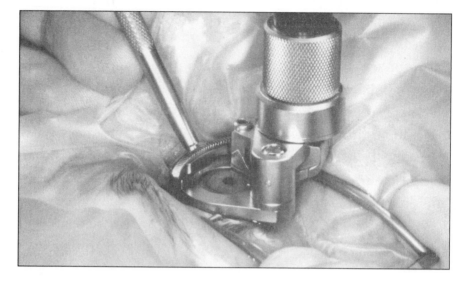

Figure 20

The Hansatome microkeratome used to create the protective corneal flap during the LASIK procedure. A microkeratome is an electromechanically controlled surgical instrument that works rather like a miniature carpenter's plane with a finely honed blade locked in its metal jaws.

(Reproduced with permission from Bausch & Lomb Surgical courtesy of Lucio Buratto, M.D., as presented in the "Down Up LASIK with the New Chiron Microkeratome.")

To answer these questions and to help you understand what it's like to have LASIK eye surgery, let's follow Karen as her corneal surgeon strives to correct her nearsighted, non-dominant eye to 20/40 from -10 diopters (which is off the chart). Since she has age-related presbyopia, Dr. Slade will slightly undercorrect this eye. If he leaves it a little nearsighted, Karen will be able to focus better up close and may be able to read a menu without reading glasses. Next week, he will try to bring her dominant eye as close to 20/20 as possible—without overcorrecting her (making her farsighted).

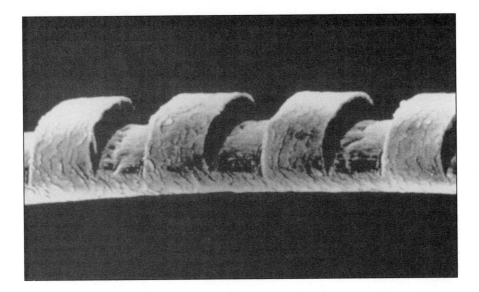

Figure 21
Human hair etched by the extremely precise excimer laser.

Picture this sober surgical scenario. Covered with clean sheets to keep her warm in the icy, humidity-controlled operating suite, Karen is lying on her back in a darkened room with her head under the laser. Every strand of her curly hair is hidden under her blue surgical cap. The same magnified image of Karen's brown eye that Dr. Slade sees through the operating microscope appears on a TV monitor in the upper corner of the operating room.

Wearing no perfume or mascara (scent affects the laser optics and mascara can get in the surgical field), she is about to undergo the initial, critical step of what is basically a two-part operation. During the first half of the LASIK procedure, the "keratectomy" (*kerato* means "cornea" and *ectomy* means to "excise," or cut), Dr. Slade will create the protective hinged flap from Karen's cornea. This round, paper-thin living tissue—which lacks refractive power—will remain attached to her peripheral cornea—rather like this page is connected to this book.

During the last five minutes of the procedure—called the laser "photoablation" by ophthalmologists—Karen's eyesight literally will be refocused by the light. Dr. Slade will lift the newly created flap and use the cool laser light scalpel to "zap" or remove tissue from the middle layer of her cornea. As you now know, this will change the way Karen's eye refracts light. Although the multi-million dollar technology behind LASIK is mind-boggling, and the pre-surgical set-up requires meticulous attention to detail, Karen's entire operation will take less than ten minutes. Karen's doctor has performed tens of thousands of LASIK operations, and he always methodically follows a surgical "pre-flight" check list.

With optometrist Dr. Richard N. Baker and an ophthalmology fellow at his side, Dr. Slade begins by gently covering Karen's face with a plastic drape. It looks like a clear mask with a hole cut out for her eye. The surgeon carefully tucks every eyelash under the plastic to provide a clear path for the disposable, surgical blade housed in the tiny microkeratome. To ensure that she doesn't blink at the wrong time and that her eyelids and "conjunctiva" (the delicate membrane covering the white of the eye) are out of the way, Karen's doctor skillfully tucks titanium specula (lid retractors) under her eyelids. As her doctor expands the specula to hold her eyelids open for maximum operating exposure, Karen's soft brown eye bulges between the metal wires, which are locked in position. Even though this sounds painful, she doesn't seem to mind. Dr. Baker has given her a sedative such as Valium to relax her and has put topical anesthetic drops in her surgically clean eye to prevent pain. Antibiotic drops and the sterilizing effects of the ultraviolet excimer laser beam will help protect her from infection.

"Karen, your job—and it is an extremely important one—is to look straight ahead at the red light," says Dr. Slade.

Holding a vacuum suction ring that looks rather like a tiny metal washer, Dr. Slade is getting ready to raise the pressure inside the globe of Karen's anesthetized eye (see fig. 18a). To do this, he must apply just the right amount of suction to her eye. So after double-checking the suction gauge and feeling the pull of the pump by holding his thumb under the ring, Dr. Slade centers it on his patient's cornea. Now, framed by Karen's thick, draped, black eyelashes, the suction ring, which has a little geared track running along its side, will immobilize her eye, holding it perfectly still during the keratectomy. When Karen's surgeon is ready to create the protective flap, the blade-bearing microkeratome will lock into this track and move automatically along the suction ring (see fig. 18b). Essential to excellent post-surgical results, the elevated intra-ocular pressure makes the corneal tissue easier to cut.

"Karen," says Dr. Slade, "the loud noise you are about to hear is the suction pump." So that it won't startle her, he demonstrates the cracking sound of the pneumatic pump, which has a back-up power supply. "Your vision will become gray temporarily during suction," he says.

Firmly steadying Karen's anesthetized eye, Dr. Slade says: "Apply suction." As Dr. Baker presses the suction switch (it is safely taped out of the way to avoid accidental deactivation), the moist brown part of Karen's eye appears gripped by the inner circle of the metal ring.

"Are you okay, Karen?" asks Dr. Baker.

"Yes. I feel a little pressure, but no pain," mutters Karen. Although her lips aren't moving, she later says she was praying almost every second of the operation.

During the next crucial step of Karen's surgery, Dr. Slade must confirm that he is about to resect (cut) a flap that is exactly the right size. To determine that the diameter of the newly created corneal flap will be correct, the surgeon places a special, plastic magnifying lens called an "applanation lens" over Karen's cornea on the suction ring. He knows that the amount of tissue applanated will be the amount of tissue cut by the surgical blade. The flap must be large enough so that, once it is lifted, Dr. Slade can laser the correct size "optical zone" (the new treated lens-like area) on Karen's inner cornea. The diameter of her new curved lens will be important to her night vision. When Karen's pupil dilates in a darkened room to let in more light, she could experience night glare and halos if light should pass through an untreated ring-shaped area.

"I am going to check the pressure inside your eye now, Karen. You shouldn't feel anything," says Dr. Slade, reassuring her. He places a cone-shaped ophthalmic instrument called a "tonometer" on her eye. The surgeon must take this reading immediately before passing the surgical blade across Karen's cornea because he has to make absolutely certain that her intra-ocular pressure is high enough to perform a good keratectomy. If the suction is inadequate, the newer keratomes will not allow the cutting motion to begin. In such a case, the operation would be aborted.

LASIK is a microsurgical procedure in which tolerances are measured in millionths of a meter. Critical to Karen's eyesight, the cut not only must be perfectly smooth, it also must be at precisely the correct depth. So with painstaking attention to detail, the surgeon verifies that Dr. Baker has assembled the metal microkeratome properly. Both of Karen's doctors listen to the sound of its motor, which is about half the length of a penlight. To make an even cut, the tiny machine must drive the keratome and its oscillating blade at a perfectly constant rate of speed.

As the surgical team checks and rechecks every part of the finely calibrated microkeratome, they pay special attention to two key parts—the beveled blade and the "depth-plate." Dr. Slade always uses a new blade for each patient. He knows that its sharp edge is flawless because he has examined it under the microscope. A surgeon must never fail to confirm that both the blade and the depth-plate—which together set the depth of the cut—are securely seated in the keratome. There is no room for error here! These two parts determine the all-important thickness of the cap-like flap and the remaining corneal bed.

Dr. Slade is using an advanced model microkeratome with special safety features, including internal diagnostics to ensure system integrity. Its electronics prevent it from working unless the suction is good. The new keratome, which has a fixed depth plate, has a capacitor in a hydraulic box so that, if the electrical power goes off, the surgeon can complete the procedure.

A "bandage" of living tissue, the flap will protect the middle layers of Karen's cornea from exposure to the air after the laser treatment. This transparent sliver of corneal tissue must be thick enough to avoid "irregular astigmatism" (a fine irregular wrinkling of the corneal surface). The more skilled the doctor, the less likely it is that this rare complication will occur. If improperly handled, a slightly damaged flap can lead to lost lines of vision on the eye chart—even with glasses. To promote visual stability, the remaining corneal layer (doctors call it the residual "stromal" bed) under the flap must be at least as thick as two pages of this book.

"Everything is going well, Karen," says the doctor. "I am almost ready to perform the keratectomy." Right before the cut, he wets the cornea with drops of buffered saline solution to avoid producing a painful corneal abrasion. At all times, he must control the hydration status of the eye. If Karen's cornea becomes too dry, she could be overcorrected. If it is too hydrated, she might be undercorrected.

Dr. Slade now places the automated microkeratome over Karen's cornea. The surgeon hooks the sharp instrument into the geared track that runs along the suction ring. Looking through the microscope, he thoroughly inspects the surgical field one last time. After only a moment's hesitation, he places his foot above the forward keratome footpedal. (It works like a car accelerator; it runs only when the foot is on the pedal.) He presses it. As the microkeratome skims smoothly across the surface of Karen's anesthetized eye, the blade cuts a paper-thin protective flap. A pre-set "stopper" on the instrument stops the blade dead in its tracks before it can resect the whole cap, leaving the flap attached on one edge of the cornea. The entire cut takes only about three seconds.

"Release suction," says Dr. Slade. With a deliberate flip of his wrist, Dr. Baker's hand hits the suction pump switch.

"Perfect," says Dr. Slade. "I am removing the suction ring from your eye, Karen. Now I want you to stare at the red aiming beam for me."

The doctor notes that Karen has good fixation. Then in one elegant motion, he skillfully lifts the flap from the corneal surface with special forceps and lays the newly cut living tissue on the white of Karen's eye. The glistening cut surface of Karen's grainy inner cornea now appears on the TV monitor. Every second counts now. The faster her doctor can sculpt her delicate corneal bed and get the flap back in place, the better Karen's eye will look tomorrow. If the fragile flap wrinkles or becomes sticky, and the surgeon fails to smooth it out, the quality of Karen's vision will be adversely affected.

"The flap looks great, Karen," says Dr. Slade, reassuring her. He is almost ready to proceed to the second half of Karen's high-tech LASIK procedure—the laser treatment of her nearsightedness and astigmatism. Doctors call this part of the surgery the "submicron photoablation of the newly exposed corneal bed." With exacting precision, the laser's cool ultraviolet beam will remove microscopic layers of tissue with minimal damage to the surrounding area. Thus, the excimer "light blade" will reshape Karen's cornea, causing it to flatten. Images will then be focused on her retina instead of in front of it.

At the beginning of Karen's surgery, Dr. Slade asked her to spell her last name and to give her date of birth. He typed all the pertinent information about Karen's case into the computer that drives the laser. These pivotal facts, including her refraction and a profile of the diameter of the ablation (the area to be lasered), now appear on the Patient Data Screen (fig. 22). Dr. Slade, Dr. Baker, and the ophthalmology fellow each have checked every number against Karen's color-coded patient chart.

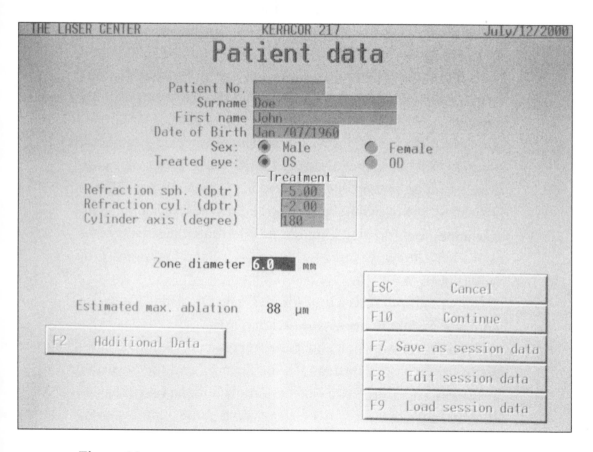

Figure 22

The patient data computer screen on the excimer laser. The patient's refraction (the spherical power to reduce near- or farsightedness and the axis of astigmatism) and the profile of the diameter of the "ablation," or laser treatment, appear on the screen of the computer that controls the excimer laser. Under direction from the doctor, the computer causes the laser to remove tissue from the cornea to improve vision.

An important point: Karen's surgical results will depend not only on an excellent keratectomy to make the flap and on the precise calibration of the laser, but also on her surgeon's "corneal math," or his "operative correction codes." Absolutely critical to how well Karen will be able to see, these mathematically derived surgical tables (doctors call them "nomograms") will determine the exact diameter and thickness of the tissue that the laser will remove from Karen's exposed inner cornea. With his usual obsessive attention to every minute detail, Dr. Slade has customized his computer-controlled laser and his operative tables to the LASIK procedure and to his personal surgical style.

"I am almost ready to treat your eye with the laser. It won't hurt, Karen," says Dr. Slade, as he gently adjusts the position of her head and carefully centers the laser over her visual axis, or line-of-sight. "Keep staring at the red fixation light for me," her doctor coaxes, as he looks at the surgical field with the high magnification of the operating microscope. Reflected in his patient's eye, the surgeon can see the two white microscope lights, the red fixation light, and the red laser focusing beam. As he fine-tunes the latter, a technician assistant gently picks up Karen's left hand and holds it to comfort her.

"Karen, can you relax a little for me?" asks Dr. Slade. "The noise that you are about to hear is the excimer laser."

Before Karen was put under the microscope, Dr. Slade carefully tested the laser's cutting rate, or "fluence," and the purity, or "homogeneity," of the beam pattern. Simply put, the laser's fluence will determine the amount of tissue each pulse removes from Karen's eye. The beam's homogeneity indicates the degree of uniformity throughout its tiny vaporizing footprint.

"Now, look at the red aiming light, Karen. Look at one point on the light. That's great!" he says, concentrating on the centration beams to keep Karen's eye centered under the laser's focal point. As he activates the laser with the foot pedal, noisy laser pulses echo around the operating room. Karen continues to stare at the light. "Perfect. Perfect. Perfect. Hold it," says Dr. Slade; the sound of his soothing voice softens the harsh staccato clicking of the machine.

With the first laser zap, the treatment screen displayed on the colored monitor suddenly springs to life. Counting rapidly backward throughout the vaporization of the tissue, the computer causes the laser to fire shot after shot during the pre-treatment, each of three ablation zones, and the astigmatic treatment. As each zone is lasered, a bright blue bar advances across the red screen showing the progress of her treatment. The surgical technician calls out the number of remaining laser pulses to Karen's doctors.

The computer's sophisticated software is guiding the laser's photoablative beam across Karen's inner cornea, following the instructions that her doctor has entered into the machine's terminal. To reduce myopia, more laser energy strikes the center of the treated area than the peripheral portion, thereby removing a curved lens-shaped volume of tissue from the middle layer of the cornea. On a cellular level, the excimer laser breaks targeted chemical bonds within the stroma's (the middle layer's) bed. Each invisible laser pulse removes only a quarter of a micron. For comparison, a minuscule red blood cell is a whopping seven microns in diameter. Such unbelievable precision helps keep the window of Karen's eye transparent.

"Keep your eyes perfectly still," says the surgeon, continuing to hold Karen's head with his hands. "I'll move your head. Don't move. That's super." Any time Karen loses fixation on the light, Dr. Slade instantly stops the laser treatment by taking his foot off the switch that activates the laser.

If Karen had been unable to keep her gaze on the red aiming light, her doctor could have stabilized the globe of her eye with surgical sponges or small forceps. In some cases, he uses an eye-tracking system to help guide the laser. Based on "Star Wars" technology, the eye tracker automatically follows radical and involuntary microscopic eye movements. Using a high resolution infrared video camera and advanced parallel processing, the computer's "laser radar" locks onto the image of the pupil.

In between each ablation, or treatment, zone, Dr. Slade gently wipes a soft surgical sponge across her inner cornea to keep it from becoming too wet. Since this fragile middle layer of cornea is exposed to the air, Karen's surgeon moves with practiced speed.

"Don't move. We are about to treat your astigmatism now," Dr. Slade says. He is holding the putter-like spatula over the underside of the hinged flap to protect it from the laser beam. Once again, he puts a drop of saline solution on the flap to keep it from becoming dehydrated. In Karen's case, Dr. Slade treats her astigmatism after her nearsightedness, but he usually does the astigmatic correction first.

"You're one of my best patients, Karen. Your laser treatment went well. Now, continue to hold perfectly still for me," Dr. Slade says, as he expertly lays the flap back on Karen's corneal bed. Since her doctor doesn't want any lint or other tiny debris between the flap and the lasered area, he irrigates underneath the repositioned flap with a special syringe. In this way, the flap is "floated" back into its natural position so that it can mold itself to the reshaped inner cornea.

"Your eye looks great, Karen," says Dr. Slade, as he carefully examines the surgical field through the microscope. He must verify that the flap is perfectly centered. The surgeon knows that the flap must not be wrinkled in any manner! So with great care, he repeatedly soothes the repositioned tissue into the newly treated stromal bed with a moistened surgical sponge.

Now Karen's surgeon puts a tiny drop of buffered saline solution in the exact center of the flap. The fluid never touches the flap's edges, which must dry for a couple of minutes.

Dr. Slade knows that his patient will be able to see better the day after surgery if he keeps the center moist and the edges relatively dry.

"I am checking the circular edge of the flap to make certain that its entire surface has adhered to the bed of your cornea. It looks fine, Karen."

"We are almost finished," says Dr. Slade. He carefully removes the lid specula and plastic drape and re-examines her eye with the microscope.

"Blink for me a couple of times," says Dr. Slade, looking through the microscope to verify that the flap is still secure. No stitches are required because the repositioned tissue is held in place by the adhesive force of capillary attraction (rather as a contact lens adheres to the eye) and by the inward sucking action of tiny metabolic "pumps" inside the cornea.

"You did great!" says Dr. Slade, as he puts drops in her newly refocused eye to promote healing and to help prevent infection. Although Karen's cornea is flatter, it is still basically convex in shape. She sits up.

"We don't want you to get hit in the eye—not even with water, Karen," says Dr. Baker. To protect her eye while she is sleeping, he gives her a clear plastic shield to wear at night.

"I can't believe how fast that was," says Karen, as the attending ophthalmology fellow helps her from the operating table to her husband's side in the post-surgical waiting area.

After her eye settles down, Karen is put in an examining room. As he looks at her eye with the slit-lamp microscope, Dr. Baker tells Karen that her cornea looks good. Glancing at the TV-like monitor, she can see a frozen image of her cornea as it appears to her doctor under magnification.

Fearing that pain lurks only moments away, Karen asks, "Will Dr. Slade prescribe a pain-killer in case my eye aches after the anesthetic eye drops wear off?"

"Does your eye hurt now?" asks Dr. Baker.

"No, but I'm afraid it will."

"Most patients don't need pain mediation after this surgery," says Dr. Baker, "but we can give you a prescription in case you need it."

Staring at Karen's eye, her husband says, "It's uncanny. Aside from a little redness and some tearing, I'd never know that you just had eye surgery."

While her husband drives her home from the clinic, Karen says, "The numbers are a little blurry, but I think that I can read the license plate on the car directly ahead of us. Before surgery I could hardly see the car without glasses," she exclaims with a huge smile."

Striving to keep the body's inflammatory response to a minimum, the LASIK surgeon must expose the inner cornea, reshape it, and close the flap quickly. For Karen this will mean that on postoperative day one, her eye—which will show no obvious signs of having had surgery—should provide good vision.

THE RECOVERY

Upon returning home, Karen's eye feels slightly scratchy. Some of the solutions used at the time of surgery can irritate the tissues, causing a slight burning sensation. She has a little more discomfort than most patients because her eyes are extremely dry. Her tear film is barely adequate to lubricate her cornea properly. Since her refractive error was severe, her laser treatment required many more pulses than the majority of patients. Although few LASIK patients take pain medication, Karen swallows one pill and goes to sleep.

Awakening about four hours later, she flips on the Food Channel from her bed. To her amazement, she can see the TV with no glasses. "The colors are spectacular!" she exclaims to her husband, who is working at his desk. "If I concentrate, I can even read the writing at the bottom of the screen." Her eye feels better—only a little gritty.

Early the next morning Karen returns to her doctors' office.

Dr. Baker examines the surface of her eye with corneal video topography. He can see that the curvature of her cornea is flatter than before her LASIK procedure.

Next, he looks at her eye through the slit-lamp microscope. Once again, a picture of her magnified cornea appears on a TV-like monitor. "Health-wise, your eye looks good, Karen. The flap is set-tling down." He notes an ever-so-slight wrinkling of the tissue near the edge of the flap near her nose that doesn't affect her vision. The area over her visual axis, or line-of-sight, is clear. "What is your impression of your vision?"

"It is pretty amazing. I actually feel younger. I feel free—it's almost like being eight years old again. My only complaint, Dr. Baker, is that I seem to be looking through a slight mist."

"It should clear up in a matter of days," Dr. Baker says. "The day after surgery, the cornea is still a little swollen. How does your eye feel?"

"It feels fine except that it is watery—but yet so dry."

"Your eye is watery in response to the surgery. Lubricating eye drops should help the dryness," the doctor explains, handing her a sample.

"The drops you gave me earlier make my eyes burn a little," Karen tells him.

"I want you to continue to use the antibiotic drops because the risk of infection is still there. If they burn too much, let us know. We have someone on call twenty-four hours a day."

As he highlights the 20/50 line, Dr. Baker then asks, "Can you identify any of the figures on this line of the eye chart, Karen?"

"Yes," Karen says, reading the letters. "I can even see some of the letters on the line below, but they are fuzzy. Why are the figures a little hazy?"

"It's part of the healing process. Your vision should become clearer over time, depending on your individual reaction to the surgery." Dr. Baker adds, "Although the flap has natural adhesive properties, Karen, I still don't want you to get hit in the eye—not with a finger, a makeup applicator, nor a tree branch."

"I want to go ahead and schedule surgery for my other eye," Karen says as she leaves the examining room.

Pain often keeps us from hurting ourselves. But Karen feels so good at home that she starts to pick up a forty-pound potted plant. Feeling the pressure of the weight in her head, she instantly stops herself. I am only one day post-op, she thinks. But the damage has already been done. When she looks in the mirror, she sees a bright red blood-filled area about the size of a nickel on the right side of the white of her eye. Terrified, Karen grabs the phone to call her doctors. Dr. Baker tells her to come to the office right away.

After examining her eye, Dr. Baker says, "Your eye will be all right. You have a subconjunctival hemorrhage. Rather like a bruise, it may get worse or change color, but it should resolve itself with time—in about three or four weeks. It won't affect your surgical result."

With every passing day, Karen's vision improves. Within two months, she can read the 20/30 line of the eye chart with both eyes, and she no longer complains of misty or hazy vision. Her close-up eyesight is the last thing to improve. For several months, Karen wears magnifying glasses when she works at her desk.

"My eyes still feel a little dry and tired when I read," Karen tells Dr. Slade.

"When your eyes are tired, your whole body feels that way. Patients often mention that their eyes are more dry or sensitive during the healing phase when there is more metabolic activity.

Your result, however, depends on the final curvature of your cornea. You won't harm your eyes by using them. Your near vision should get better, but, even though you have surgically-induced monovision, you will probably still need magnifiers to read the newspaper."

And that is exactly what happened. Eventually, Karen would be fairly pleased with her near vision—her new eyesight from about one foot to about seven feet away. This is the range that people lose in their forties. It is frustrating to search for glasses in order to change the reading on your air-conditioning thermostat. It is even more irritating to look through trifocal lines to glance from your plate to your friend to the doorway.

As Karen told Dr. Slade, "The thing that I'm most thrilled about is my increased range of vision." She added laughing, "I still need a magnifying mirror to see my wrinkles—but that may be an advantage."

Some LASIK patients feel a little too good for the safety of their eyes. Doctors know how to react to the variables that can occur during the actual LASIK operation, but we have no control of what our patients do when they leave our office—and yet, in a way, we feel responsible for them. We have had people go jogging two days after surgery. Worse yet, one extremely athletic patient, a thirty-three-year-old executive with a -5 diopter correction, went skiing in the Rocky Mountains three days after having LASIK on both eyes.

"I felt fine," he told me later.

"That is a bit much," I said, trying to be tactful.

"I skied better than ever, even though my vision fluctuated slightly. The wind blowing around my sun glasses made my eyes a little dry," he added.

Even the brightest people don't always use their common sense. I was exceedingly grateful that he didn't get hit in the eye with a ski pole or a hot dogger's elbow.

THE MUNNERLYN FORMULA: THE MATHEMATICAL SAFETY NET

If you decide to have LASIK or PRK, the calculations that determine your future eyesight will be based on a mathematical equation called the Munnerlyn formula. It ensures that the window of your eye has enough remaining corneal tissue underneath the newly sculpted lens to maintain the stability of the cornea. A crucial amount of the stroma, the main inner corneal layer, and the last two layers must remain intact. Developed by famous California physicist Dr. Charles Munnerlyn, the formula described in the medical equation, states:

The depth of the treatment zone (the thickness of the lens) =
[the diameter of the lens (the treated zone) in millimeters² x the
number of diopters of correction] / 3

In effect, this formula means that the wider the diameter of your lens—and the greater your refractive error—the deeper your surgeon must laser into your cornea to correct your vision. Put another way, the larger the diameter of your optical zone and the more nearsighted you are, the more corneal tissue the laser must remove (see the Appendix on page 271 for more on the Munnerlyn Formula). Ophthalmologists sometimes simply say that the depth of the laser treatment is proportional to the size of the optical zone. This means that, depending on your correction, the wider your new lens, the thicker it must be. Of course, to treat nearsightedness, more laser light strikes the center of the cornea, thereby removing more tissue there than from the periphery. A small increase in the diameter of this curved optical zone causes a significant increase in the amount of the corneal tissue removed. Nevertheless, even a -6 diopter correction with a 6-millimeter optical zone only vaporizes 72 microns of tissue.

Your doctor will want you to look through a large optical zone that is about 6 millimeters in diameter. A wide, finely sculpted corneal lens is especially important for good night vision when the pupil dilates to let in more light. As the pupil widens beyond the lasered area for patients with a small optical zone, the light coming through the untreated edge of the cornea is unfocused. Severely nearsighted people often have large pupils. When the diameter of the uncorrected lens is too small for the size of the dilated pupil, the ring-shaped part of the cornea that remains "nearsighted" can cause halos around lights at night. Patients find this phenomenon extremely distracting. Physicians now have computer software that allows them to re-treat patients with this problem to make their optical zones larger.

THE EXCIMER LASER: THE KEY TO MODERN REFRACTIVE SURGERY

The cool excimer laser, the most technologically advanced surgical tool to treat refractive errors, has revolutionized vision correction surgery (see fig. 23). This remarkably precise ultraviolet laser creates invisible pulses of light that remove microscopic amounts of corneal tissue. Controlled by customized software, a computer calculates the number of laser shots required to achieve a patient's targeted refraction.

The excimer laser can be delivered in various ways. The older broad-beam lasers have about a 7-millimeter footprint that is partially masked by a diaphragm. As it opens, expanding outward from the center, the diameter of the beam that reaches the cornea increases. This means that the center of the nearsighted cornea receives the most treatment, leaving the edges tapered. The newer flying-spot, or scanning, lasers with small beam footprints emit less energy per pulse than the broad-beam machines (see fig. 24). The

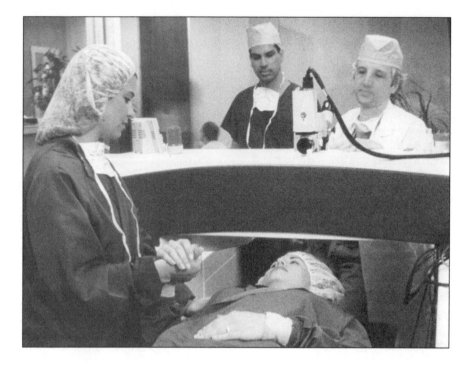

Figure 23
Dr. Slade (far right) performing LASIK.

computer programs tell the scanning mirrors within the laser exactly how to move to aim the beam and how many pulses to emit at a specific location. As the scanning beam moves back and forth across the cornea, the laser creates a smoother recontoured surface than the older lasers. These advanced machines also should improve refractive predictability.

In the 1970s, IBM scientists, experimenting with different gas mixtures to create new lasers, found that the 193-nanometer wavelength of laser energy can remove molecules of tissue with little damage to the surrounding area. (One nanometer equals one billionth of a meter.) Now known as the excimer laser, this wavelength is so exact that it can cut notches in a human hair and etch tiny microcircuits into computer chips (see fig. 21). Used as a light

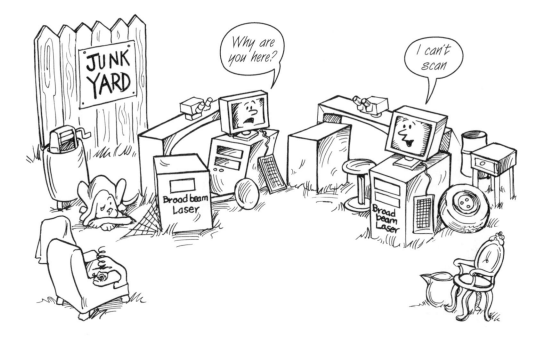

Figure 24
Old laser junk yard.

scalpel, the excimer reacts with protein molecules, breaking molecular bonds. "Photoablating"—vaporizing corneal tissue at the submicron level (a micron is one millionth of a meter)—the excimer's short pulses penetrate to an exact and predictable depth. With unfathomable speed, each laser pulse can remove 39 millionths of an inch of tissue in 12 billionths of a second. Such extraordinary accuracy helps doctors achieve excellent control over the amount of tissue removed during the procedure.

How does a laser work? Briefly, *laser* stands for "light amplification by stimulated emission of radiation." Laser light is created when energy is applied to a mixture of gases. Two gaseous elements such as argon and fluoride in a helium premix are jolted to a higher energy state with thousands of volts of electricity. These elements combine to form an unstable compound. As the excited ionized atoms dance within a mirrored tube that reflects the light back at them, they release an intense concentration of light energy. Eventually, the light beam becomes so energized that part of it escapes from the tube through a hole in the semi-silvered mirror. Such laser light—unlike sunlight—is focused in one direction at one wavelength. In other words, the light rays vibrate together in phase to form a "coherent" monochromatic laser beam.

The essential point for patients to understand about the excimer laser is that their doctor needs to grasp fully all the intricacies of how the instrument works. A surgeon must know how the characteristics of the laser beam are affected by its environment— by temperature and humidity—and how the device is tested or calibrated before each surgery. Even the altitude of the clinic affects results and is factored into the mathematical formulas that control the excimer. Lasers are not static instruments. They are constantly changing. Replacing a lens in the optical system or replenishing the laser's gases affects the characteristics of the beam.

Ophthalmologists would never perform radial keratotomy (RK) for nearsightedness without knowing the exact length and quality of the diamond blade. Nor would they make an incision in a patient's cornea with a diamond that has a chip in it. Similarly, a corneal laser surgeon must never perform LASIK or PRK without knowing the cutting, or "ablation," rate and quality of the excimer's beam. Hence, the physician has to monitor continually the laser's "fluence" (ablation or vaporization rate) and its "homogeneity" (the uniformity of the footprint, or pattern, of the beam). No part of the beam's footprint should cut much deeper than any other part. This means that the laser must be recalibrated before each patient.

Rather as a fine violin should be tuned before every symphony, an excimer laser must be carefully tested before each procedure. The violin's pitch can shift ever so slightly with each stroke of the bow. The profile of the laser beam varies minutely with every pulse.

Like the violinist, the surgeon must know that the laser is "in tune" so that it can perform well.

Some patients worry that any one laser pulse might negatively affect the final outcome. With a great painting, no single, tiny brush stroke brings the final picture to life. With refractive laser surgery, no one laser pulse has a noticeable effect on your ultimate vision. In fact, the slight, natural micro-movements of the eye add to a blending or polishing effect. Rather as the accumulation of many delicate brush strokes creates a Rembrandt's poignant emotional impact, the sum of a pre-set number of laser pulses produces the joy of finely sculpted vision.

THE FUTURE: CUSTOM LASIK

After having the high-tech LASIK procedure, many patients see almost as well without glasses as they did beforehand with them. But even though doctors are getting excellent outcomes using today's sophisticated lasers and computer software, we continue to strive for even better results. The ultimate dream of refractive surgery is to fine-tune patients' vision *beyond* what they currently have with glasses or contacts. Toward this end, a recent breakthrough in LASIK surgery based on "wavefront" technology (think of the edge of an ocean wave applied to light) is showing extremely promising early results.

Currently, doctors are basing LASIK treatments on what patients tell them during an eye exam. In other words, each eye's refractive error is largely determined by how you answer the question: "Which is better, one or two?" as you sit behind the dial-up phoropter lenses looking at the eye chart. With this subjective method of measuring focusing errors, all patients with a -2 diopter correction have the same number entered in the laser's computer. But just because you and a friend both have a -2 diopter refraction doesn't mean that your eyes are exactly alike. In truth, the prescription ground into your glasses is only part of the story of how your eyes focus light.

Most LASIK patients are fairly happy if their post-surgical visual acuity is as good as their pre-surgical vision with soft contact lenses. But with the new custom wavefront LASIK, we may be able to tell patients: "After surgery you probably won't need glasses, and—depending on how you heal—you might even see *better* than you now do with your glasses or soft contacts."

With custom wavefront LASIK, the surgical treatment, which is called the "laser ablation" by doctors, is personalized to the individual. Detailed information about the patient's optical system is fed into the computer. With this data, the incredibly sophisticated scanning laser—under the surgeon's watchful eye—can sculpt your cornea to a more perfect form.

To understand how custom LASIK works, let's first consider another advanced technique called "topographic LASIK." For years, doctors scanned the *front surface* of the cornea to map its topography or shape. More recently, surgeons have been able to use this surface information to guide "topo-linked" scanning lasers. Now, by using the even more sophisticated topography systems, we can peer deeper into your eyes to study how they refract light. This technology not only shows the height and curvature of the front of your cornea but also the back. In addition, such maps illustrate corneal depth and that of the anterior chamber and produce a refractive model of your eye that can be linked (like "topo-linked") to the laser's computer. It can learn from previous operations on other patients, although it still is unable to adjust instantly for its changes in real time. This wonderful technology enables us to correct people who have less-than-optimal refractive surgery outcomes—for example, persons with irregular astigmatism or decentered ablations (incorrectly placed laser treatments).

The new custom LASIK based on wavefront technology even goes a step beyond topography-linked LASIK. By adding ultrasound and light-ray tracing, the doctor can scan your eye's structures and draw more detailed maps. To test objectively the eye's total focusing power, wavefront analysis uses light and ray tracing to track light going into and out of the eye. The retina's curved surface reflects and even refracts light. Since none of us has a perfect optical system, our eyes create "aberrations" (distortions) in the waves of light that reach our retinas. This blurs images. They are distorted by imperfections not only in the surfaces of the front and back of your cornea, but also by irregularities on the front and back surfaces of your lens and those in the curve of your retina. So if we shine a rapidly scanning spot into your eye, a specially programmed computer, which knows the angle and characteristics of the light going in, can analyze how each tiny ray is shifted to the left, to the right, or up and down. Special wavefront sensors measure the shape of the distorted wave of light coming from the eye. In this way, the software can analyze how your eye's structures refract light.

But how can all this digitized personal data about your eyes lead to improved LASIK results? During an incredibly high-tech procedure, the excimer laser treats the cornea to compensate for the light-scattering effects of the imperfections in your eye's focusing mechanism. Once the computer analyzes your eye's total refractive power, the software produces highly accurate acuity maps. Using this data, the programs create a simulation of your best acuity and customize the correct "contour-ablation-pattern" (the laser treatment) to imprint on your eye's window. The laser's scanning beam then flies around most of your cornea, surgically changing it to counteract focusing problems. Early scientific studies seem to show that such individualized treatments offer great hope for clearer, aberration-free vision.

WHAT COULD GO WRONG?

The ten-minute LASIK procedure is so quick that it looks easy to perform. In fact, after you watch this operation four or five times in your doctor's office, you might wonder if you couldn't do it. But don't be deceived. A delicate surgery, LASIK has many fine nuances that ophthalmologists must thoroughly grasp to avoid rare intra-operative and post-operative complications. As Karen's operation illustrates, LASIK surgeons must follow a "pre-flight" checklist to prevent rare but serious problems. To avert potential difficulties, physicians must have a complete understanding of the mechanisms that cause them. In the unlikely event of an emergency, doctors must know exactly how to intervene. Fortunately, most complications can be managed immediately or at least diminished by a second operation.

Eye doctors divide refractive surgery complications into those that occur during the operation and those that arise afterward. Let's look first at the rare intra-operative complications—nearly all of which can be prevented with the latest equipment and with proper surgical technique. In the past, the most unthinkable problem that could occur during LASIK was that the blade of the small metal microkeratome might cut clear through the cornea and enter the eye's anterior chamber. This worst case scenario—which had to be avoided at all cost—demanded immediate intervention by the surgeon. A little slit could be quickly stitched shut, but if the blade pierced the crystalline lens, it had to be replaced by an artificial intra-ocular lens. With the older keratome surgical instruments, this devastating complication was avoided by triple-checking the equipment and by carefully measuring and remeasuring the thickness of the cornea. Nowadays, with the latest microkeratome called the Hansatome (see fig. 20)—which cannot perforate a normal healthy cornea—the risk of this feared intra-operative complication is eliminated.

Once the protective flap is cut, the tension in the surgical suite drops precipitously. Most of the possible serious intra-operative LASIK complications are associated with the cutting of this thin, corneal tissue. In the rare instance where the flap is improperly cut, the surgeon usually can place it back on the eye because the bottom surface of the flap matches the top of the residual stromal bed, or middle layer, of the cornea. Unless the bed is lasered or the flap position is disturbed, any irregularities in the two facing surfaces represent almost perfect templates to each other. In such a case, the surgery is aborted without proceeding to the laser treatment. In three or four months, the cornea should heal almost back to its original state. At this time, the doctor can repeat the procedure. After a new flap is made, the laser treatment usually can be performed with the patient's original post-surgical prognosis intact.

Irregular Astigmatism

By skillfully handling the flap, your doctor can minimize any fine wrinkling of this delicate tissue that scatters the light rays, leading to irregular astigmatism. Immediately after LASIK, some patients may experience slightly blurry vision from this problem, but it disappears during the normal healing process as the flap settles down. In rare cases in which irregular astigmatism fails to resolve spontaneously, the patient may lose lines of best-corrected visual acuity—that is, lose the ability to read the bottom one to three lines on the eye chart. In some cases, vision improves with time. Re-treatment with customized wavefront LASIK using the latest scanning lasers may reduce this problem. By lasering the peaks and leaving the valleys alone, the new fast lasers can smooth out some rough places. However, even with the most current technology now under study, no doctor can promise to eliminate irregular astigmatism totally.

A "Free Cap"

Your doctor must know how to manage a "free cap" (one with no hinge), even though the new keratome has greatly reduced the likelihood that this problem may occur. If this small surgical device does cut clear through the hinge, detaching the cap, it must be stored in a special chamber to control hydration during the laser treatment. After the ablation, the doctor simply places the cap back on the eye. A stitch is seldom necessary. The eye's natural suction and the regrowth of the epithelium—not the hinge—hold the cap to the corneal bed. For a patient under the care of an experienced corneal surgeon, a free cap should not adversely affect the final outcome. By careful attention to detail, the surgeon can avoid injuring or losing the cap. In the unlikely event that the cap is destroyed or lost, the doctor has two options: first, if the remaining cornea is thick enough, he can proceed with the laser treatment and then let the epithelium grow back over the newly ablated surface. Like PRK patients, these people will lose Bowman's membrane, the second layer of the cornea. Although some of them develop haze requiring further treatment, amazingly enough, most see 20/40 or better. The second option is for the surgeon to perform a "homoplastic" graft with human corneal donor tissue, which is basically a partial corneal transplant (see page 248 for detailed information on corneal transplants).

"Hot Spots" in the Laser Beam

Another complication to be avoided: the laser's tiny vaporizing footprint should not contain "hot spots" that have higher energy than the surrounding beam. To prevent this, the surgeon must test the quality of the beam before every case. A poor quality beam can cause regular or irregular astigmatism.

LASIK surgeons can get into trouble if they try to be heroes and proceed with an operation when they should cancel it. If the doctor doesn't get the flap he wants or his laser doesn't calibrate correctly, he must have the good surgical judgment to stop the procedure. Early one Friday morning, the week before Thanksgiving, we had a whole waiting room filled with people from all over the world—many of whom had surgery on their first eye the previous day. Most had reservations to fly home that Saturday. Unfortunately, when we tested the laser, the beam's quality was not up to standard. This meant that we had to send everyone home for the day. When someone's vision is at stake, the doctor must never be pressured into continuing. Part of being a good surgeon is knowing when to say, "No." If you put yourself in the right hands, even when problems occur with the equipment, your doctor will know to stop the procedure, and no harm will be done.

CENTRAL ISLANDS

Occasionally during surgery, a tiny raised area in the central part of the treated zone doesn't receive sufficient laser treatment. On topographical analysis, these steep areas look like little islands, so doctors refer to them as "central islands." Any such irregularity in the curvature of the cornea's surface affects the transmission of light and can decrease the effectiveness of the procedure. No two lasers are exactly alike. Hence, surgeons must customize their formulas, or nomograms, to each particular machine to avoid central islands. With time, central islands often shrink spontaneously. In any event, an unresolved island can usually be successfully re-treated with further surgery to remove the elevated area. The new scanning, or flying-spot, lasers have eliminated this complication, but even the original lasers have software to prevent these surface flaws.

Decentered Laser Treatment

The surgically created living "lens" must be centered directly over the patient's visual axis, or line-of-sight (see fig. 6). A perfect-placed laser treatment is especially critical when treating astigmatism. We have seen rare referred cases in which the photoablation was off center, meaning that the patient looks through the wrong part of the newly recontoured corneal lens. Called a "decentered ablation" by doctors, this avoidable problem is immediately apparent on topographic maps of the cornea. People with off-centered ablations are usually undercorrected without glasses. Their best-corrected vision also may drop because of surgically induced irregular astigmatism. In addition, these patients may complain of halos and ghost images. To avoid an off-center correction, all the optics inside the laser must be properly aligned. By pre-testing the laser, the surgeon makes absolutely certain that the invisible laser beam is coincident with the colored aiming beam. The laser light must be perfectly aligned with the surgeon's eyepiece. Even though the patient faithfully stares at the aiming beam, if it isn't aligned with the laser beam, the removal of tissue will be off center. If the patient is unable to fixate, the surgeon may have to stop the procedure. We have successfully treated referred patients with decentered optical zones by using one of the new flying-spot lasers. The new customized wavefront LASIK may help these patients.

Undercorrection

By far the most common post-operative complaint of near-sighted patients about LASIK is that they are undercorrected. In other words, they have residual myopia. An overcorrection, which means that a nearsighted patient becomes farsighted, also can occur. As we discuss in detail later, the crystalline lens of a young patient can compensate for a little farsightedness, but older people, who are unable to accommodate, are extremely unhappy if they become too farsighted. Refractive surgeons avoid this problem by slightly undercorrecting patients. A repeat laser treatment with either myopic or hyperopic LASIK may be necessary to improve the final outcome of these complications (see chapter 11 on enhancements).

The more experience your surgeon has performing LASIK, the closer she can target your outcome to 20/20—without overcorrecting you. Remember, to achieve the most accurate correction, your doctor uses computerized mathematical calculations (surgical tables) to plan your refraction. Based on results with earlier patients, these surgical tables, or nomograms, which are specially designed for LASIK (not for PRK), are customized for your physician's individual excimer laser and her surgical technique. Since your doctor updates and fine-tunes her nomograms from past experience with her laser, the tables become more accurate as the number of patients in the sample increases. As you might imagine, ophthalmologists who have performed thousands of LASIK procedures generally have more precise surgical tables than doctors who have done only a handful of operations.

All beginning LASIK surgeons must start conservatively by targeting corrections that leave patients a little nearsighted rather than farsighted. As they gain experience tracking their results, eye doctors are able to nudge their surgical corrections closer to the mark. Among experienced LASIK surgeons, significant overcorrections are uncommon. When they do occur, doctors have the technology to refocus farsightedness with hyperopic LASIK.

HALOS AND GLARE

The mysterious dark pupils that gather the light coming into your eyes are unique. Surrounded by the colored iris, pupils come in different sizes. They automatically constrict to protect your eyes from the sun. They dilate or enlarge to let more light reach the retina at night. To obtain good LASIK results, doctors must carefully measure how much your round pupils widen in the dark. To avoid halos and glare, your surgeon has to make certain that your new optical zone, the area treated by the laser, is adequate for your individual pupil size in low light conditions. In other words, your ophthalmologist must match your optical zone to the size of your pupil when it's fully dilated. Your doctor should examine your pupils with a special instrument to determine exactly how large they become at night. We use a night-vision scope like those used by the military. A few people have larger-than-average pupils that become even bigger at night. Let's say that someone's pupils dilate to a 7.5 millimeters in total darkness. If this person has LASIK, and the total post-surgical treatment zone is only 6 millimeters across, the light coming through the un-lasered area may be associated with halos and glare.

One of the advantages of the newer scanning lasers over the original broad-beam ones is that the older lasers were limited to an optical zone of about 6.5 millimeters. This size treatment zone is adequate for most people, but those with large pupils especially benefit from the scanning lasers. They can treat the approximately 11-millimeter cornea all the way out to 9 millimeters. This means that the patient will have a full correction to 6 millimeters or so and a blended zone to 9 millimeters to refract light passing through the dilated pupil at night.

If you are considering refractive surgery, you need to be aware that, even though your doctor takes every possible known precaution, some people still have glare and halos. They can be very distracting, especially if they are severe. Such problems—which are always a concern—improve with time for most patients. These complications rarely bother people after the first few months.

Keep in mind that many severely nearsighted people have glare and halos before refractive surgery. They may see the edges of their glasses or their contacts, or they may be undercorrected with their lenses. Sometimes, this problem improves after LASIK because patients' eyes are more focused. Unfortunately, some people say they still have halos afterward, but that they look different.

DISPLACED FLAP

If a LASIK patient gets hit in the eye or rubs it roughly immediately after surgery, the flap can become displaced. If the person fails to go to the doctor immediately, the gel-like epithelium will grow around and under the flap. In such a case, the surgeon must lift the flap and carefully clean the area. In rare cases, a homoplastic graft is necessary.

CORNEAL HAZE AND "HAZY" VISION

Corneal haze, which looks like a white stellar nebula under the microscope, seldom affects the vision of LASIK patients because the protective flap promotes the post-surgical healing process. Under magnification, mild, diffuse haze looks rather like fingerprints on glass. Such faint imperfections of the cornea are caused by slight disruptions in the uniformity of the arrangement of the lamellar fibers. You will recall that the natural placement of these fibers allows light wavelengths to pass through the cornea uninterrupted. Causing a temporary loss of transparency or even a slight permanent scarring, a mild dislocation of the lamellae may not be noticed by patients. A frequent complication following PRK, mild haze—which is often associated with the cornea's healing response—may resolve naturally with time. Severe cases, however, can affect visual acuity and require treatment with steroids to modulate the wound-healing response or with a repeat operation to try to reduce the haze.

Right after LASIK, patients sometimes experience noticeable swelling of the middle layer of the cornea for a brief period. These people have "hazy vision," with no apparent scarring of the cornea. This problem usually resolves naturally within two or three weeks after LASIK, although extremely nearsighted patients, especially those with dry eyes, may require a couple of months to recover from this side effect.

DRY EYES

Many patients with dry eyes seek LASIK because their contact lenses are uncomfortable. Unfortunately, after surgery their eyes may feel even drier than usual for a while. Even people with adequate tears may notice that their eyes are a little dehydrated temporarily after LASIK. Patients who have PRK are even more symptomatic than those who have LASIK.

The reason LASIK can temporarily make dry eyes feel worse is that some of the cornea's nerves are cut. They may require six to eight weeks or longer to heal before normal sensitivity returns. Even if your eyes lubricate properly before surgery, afterward— when the cornea is desensitized—you blink less. When you blink less, the cornea becomes dryer. Fortunately, most people with dry eyes are able to have LASIK even though they have more symptoms than the average surgery patient. These patients need extra care with special high-quality lubricating drops. Within a month or two, most people feel much better.

As the years pass, dry eyes tend to get worse—whether one has LASIK or not. Some people may benefit by having the lower "punctums" in their eyelids plugged. These are two of the eye's four tiny ducts that drain away your tears. When the lower ones are closed, more moisture remains in the eye. Think of closing the drain in your sink while the tap is hardly dripping. Although some people can feel the plugs in their eyes, and a few have had other problems, many of my patients feel much better after this treatment. Some can even wear contacts again.

INFECTION

With any operation, infection is always feared. With LASIK, the chance is exceedingly small, especially with antibiotic coverage. Nevertheless, this risk is with us for the first twenty-four to seventy-two hours immediately following surgery. If a patient gets an infection, and we are unable to cure it, she could permanently lose all or part of her vision. The risk of this complication is less than one in ten thousand with a highly experienced surgeon. Fortunately, most infections can be cured if treated immediately with topical antibiotics.

SANDS OF THE SAHARA

Doctors also watch for any sign of an inflammation of the cornea called the Sands of the Sahara and technically dubbed "nonspecific diffuse intralamellar keratitis" (NSDIK). A rare complication, NSDIK symptoms may vary from a mild corneal haze to an infection-like clouding that looks like swirling sand. LASIK practitioners treat mild cases with topical steroids, but severe inflammations require steroid therapy and surgical intervention. Since the "nonspecific," non-bacterial infiltrates are generally located between the flap and the residual corneal bed, the surgeon lifts the flap and cleans the interface between the two surfaces to remove the thin milky fluid. After irrigating the area, the doctor treats both surfaces with a special therapeutic laser and replaces the flap. Aggressive treatment with topical steroids follows. A good prognosis following a nonspecific inflammation of the cornea depends not only on early diagnosis and skilled intervention, but also the patient's response to the treatment.

EPITHELIAL INGROWTH

Good surgical technique can help your doctor prevent another complication called "epithelial ingrowth," whereby the gel-like corneal covering, or epithelium, grows under the flap. This problem can occur if, instead of laying the flap back in position in the correct manner, the surgeon slides the thin tissue over the epithelial cells. Proper manipulation of the flap is especially important when correcting farsightedness. As Karen's case shows, the surgeon also must take great care to smooth the edges of the flap back onto the corneal bed. If the flap fails to adhere properly, or if the edges are rough, the epithelium can creep between the two surfaces. Epithelial ingrowth, which can sometimes block vision, may be self-limiting or may require treatment.

Immediately after surgery, the physician examines the patient with the slit-lamp microscope to check that the flap is reset properly. If the surgeon finds a problem, she will re-irrigate the flap in the operating room. The ophthalmologist raises the flap and removes this debris. If left untreated, it can cause regular and irregular astigmatism, depending on the location and degree of the ingrowth. In other words, unless the misplaced epithelium is removed, it can sometimes lead to a drop in best-corrected visual acuity. In extremely rare instances in which the epithelium aggressively grows under the flap, the surgeon must act quickly to prevent corneal ulceration and infection.

REGRESSION

Unlike PRK patients, most LASIK patients do not regress. After the initial few months, the curvature of the cornea should remain reasonably stable. Mapping the cornea with computerized topography shows that the majority of LASIK patients achieve a stable refraction within the first three months after surgery. People with high myopia, however, may require six months or longer. Persons who do experience a drop in the effect of the procedure usually were severely myopic before surgery. Doctors do not know why these patients occasionally regress, but we surmise that the problem is related to the depth of the laser ablation and the healing process. The more treatment necessary, the more the stroma or middle layer of the cornea must remodel itself during the first couple of years after surgery. In addition, the epithelium may grow back a little thicker over the lasered area, especially in highly myopic patients. To overcome large amounts of nearsightedness, the laser must make a deeper ablation than to treat mild cases. The deeper the treatment, the more the body tries to fill in the depression, or "divot," with new epithelium. This natural healing response may contribute to slight-to-moderate post-surgical regression in highly myopic patients.

LASIK neither slows nor hastens the normal progression of nearsightedness. Some myopic patients, unfortunately, naturally continue to get a little more nearsighted throughout their life. If the eyeball gets slightly longer or if the crystalline lens starts to develop a cataract, the person will become more myopic even though the corneal curvature is stable. No matter how much nearsightedness naturally progresses with time, patients still should see better without glasses if they have LASIK. Consider, for example, a thirty-year-old man with -7 diopters of myopia. Over a five-year period, with or without surgery, he may naturally develop another diopter of refractive error. Without any surgery, his correction would now be -8 diopters (severe myopia). But let's say he had LASIK at thirty, and his correction was reduced to -1 diopter (mild myopia). Five years pass. His eyeball naturally elongates so that his refractive error increases to -2 diopters. At this time, he might wish to consider a re-treatment or enhancement procedure.

Scientists have noticed that people who do large volumes of close work tend to be more myopic than people who work outdoors, such as construction workers, who must focus in the distance. As you now know, when you look at a near object, your eyes converge. Pulled inward during years of reading, your eyeball could become slightly longer. An increase of only 1 millimeter in the length of the eyeball will increase myopia by as much as 3 diopters. If you squeeze a tennis ball and quickly let go, it will go back to its original shape. If you squeeze the ball sixteen hours a day for ten years, it is not unreasonable to postulate that the ball's shape could elongate slightly.

We once heard a doctor say that physicians, not patients, should worry about the complications of LASIK surgery. The implication was that, since serious problems seldom occur among experienced doctors, patients can be saved needless anxiety if they are unaware that complications can occur. We disagree. The more you know about refractive surgery, the more likely you will be to demand excellent care leading to a good result. Of course, it is impossible to include every conceivable thing that might go wrong during and after any operation. For example, one refractive surgeon had a pipe break on the floor above his laser, causing the ceiling to fall on top of the machine. Fortunately, no one was under it. In another case, when the electricity went out during an electrical storm, a doctor had to put a flap back on a patient's cornea while his assistants held emergency flash lights over the surgical field. Although the physician had his heart in his throat, the patient was totally unaware that anything was wrong and achieved excellent vision anyway.

HYPEROPIC LASIK OR H-LASIK FOR FARSIGHTEDNESS

If you are farsighted, can the new operation known as hyperopic LASIK, or "H-LASIK," improve your eyesight? Even though farsightedness is more difficult to treat than nearsightedness, and the recovery takes longer, we have achieved good results for a carefully selected group of farsighted patients. Unfortunately, hyperopic LASIK is still less accurate than refractive surgery for myopia. Some patients may take two or three months longer to achieve stable refractions following H-LASIK than following myopic LASIK. In fact, what appears to be an overcorrection after a week or even a month may become a perfect outcome after a few months' time. Generally speaking, people in the lower ranges of farsightedness attain the best visual acuity, and their results also usually are the most predictable and stable.

You will recall that to treat farsightedness with the excimer laser, the surgeon removes tissue from the mid-periphery of the cornea, creating a carefully-blended circular trench to change the curvature of the window of the eye. The goal is to make the curve of the central cornea steeper. Even though the laser is never aimed directly over the line-of-sight, the effect of surgery is over the pupil. Creating a more powerful corneal lens, hyperopic LASIK refocuses the eye so that incoming light falls on the retina instead of behind it (see figs. 5c and 11b). Depending on the outcome, refractive surgery for farsightedness can improve both near and distance vision. Nevertheless, you still probably will need reading glasses for fine print if you are over forty years old.

HOW AGE AFFECTS FARSIGHTEDNESS

Farsightedness is so named because many young people with this problem often have good distance vision. Some hyperopic patients, however, cannot see close, especially as they age. If you are farsighted, you eventually will require glasses or contact lenses when your eye's focusing mechanism no longer can place images directly on your retina. As discussed in chapter 1, as you have more birthdays, you will lose your ability to compensate for farsightedness. Over time, the crystalline lens inside the eye gradually loses its flexibility and, thus, its ability to focus close objects. Since this lens needs more power to help us read or thread a needle, farsighted people lose their near vision before their distance vision. Unfortunately, when you are in your forties, no one prescription can give you correct vision at all distances.

If your farsightedness is already affecting your driving and making your reading vision worse, refocusing your eyes with surgery should help your acuity at all distances. Typically, patients past the age of forty who have primary farsightedness along with age-related presbyopia are quite happy with their surgical results because hyperopic LASIK makes their near, mid range, and far vision better. Can refractive surgery promise to eliminate the need for magnifying mirrors and reading glasses? Unfortunately, no. But after this operation your dependence on them should be reduced. Will you be able to see your lunch, your computer, and your friends better after H-LASIK? Yes. In the best hands, your uncorrected visual acuity should improve, even though it may not be perfect.

With farsightedness, we often recommend overcorrecting one of your eyes to make it a little nearsighted. The goal is to save some of the intermediate and up-close vision for as long as possible. As with nearsighted laser treatments, monovision can reduce the strength of your reading glasses and the amount of time you need them. Accordingly, if your doctor makes you slightly nearsighted in one eye, you should be able to use it to read a menu in good light. Depending on your age, about -1 diopter of myopia could be an ideal compromise solution. Always remember that no one prescription can satisfy all your visual needs when you are over forty. Before surgery, your physician should demonstrate your targeted correction by letting you look through the phoropter lenses (the dial-up trial refractive lenses used to test your vision for glasses in his office). In addition, wearing a contact lens that makes you a little nearsighted in your non-dominant eye is an excellent way to simulate overcorrecting farsightedness in one eye. Even though farsighted corrections lack the accuracy of nearsighted ones, if hyperopic patients are past forty or so, even a partial improvement can be extremely helpful. To reiterate, when you're nearsighted, you are at least in focus at some distance. When you're farsighted and over forty, you're not in focus any place.

Who Is a Candidate for Hyperopic LASIK?

As with any refractive operation, the key issue when recommending hyperopic LASIK to someone is: Can this procedure meet this person's expectations? Since older patients with hyperopia are out of focus no matter where they look, they are much easier to please than nearsighted people. Try to imagine that you are over forty with +4 diopters of farsightedness and that you are unable to see without correction at any distance. If LASIK corrects your vision to +1 diopter, your vision won't be perfect, but you will be able to see much better. If we overcorrect you to -1 diopter, making you slightly nearsighted, you would be even happier. You at least would see clearly three feet in front of your face without glasses. In good light, you probably could even recognize friends across the room at a party. Now, if we are extremely "lucky" so that your post-surgical refractive error is -0.5 diopters, we are going to be heroes. You will have almost normal vision.

Currently, doctors can treat up to about +4 or +5 diopters of farsightedness with hyperopic LASIK. Unfortunately, we are as yet unable to correct the higher ranges of farsightedness greater than +5 or +6 diopters to our satisfaction. Doctors can make patients with high hyperopia better, but the results lack the accuracy that we would like.

If you have had refractive surgery for nearsightedness and were overcorrected so that you are now farsighted, you may be helped by H-LASIK. In other words, this operation might be able to largely compensate for a poor refractive surgery result.

With rare exceptions, we generally don't treat farsighted patients under age forty with hyperopic LASIK because they usually can still see well in the distance. Perhaps they have +3 diopters of hyperopia, but they don't "wear" it because their crystalline lens can focus without fatigue or eye strain. With our present technology, if the laser correction isn't right on target, H-LASIK can actually make a young patient's distance vision worse. For this reason, we tell people under forty: "Come back when you can no longer pass your driver's test without glasses. Then you might be a good candidate. As your crystalline lens gradually loses its ability to make up for your farsightedness, and we get better at treating hyperopia, the day may come when we'll be able help you." Currently, even the best doctors using the most advanced surgical techniques aren't good enough to promise totally accurate results.

THE H-LASIK SURGICAL PROCEDURE

In some ways, surgery for farsightedness is similar to the correction of nearsightedness—even though the laser is controlled by totally different software. Both microsurgical operations require the creation of a protective flap and the removal of tissue with the excimer light scalpel. And both surgeries are subtraction procedures, although much more tissue is removed to correct farsightedness than nearsightedness. Recall that to make the center of the cornea of the hyperopic eye steeper, the surgeon must remove tissue near the periphery. With myopic and hyperopic LASIK, the surgeon lasers to the same depth, for the same number of diopters. But, as mentioned earlier, to treat farsightedness, a much larger area is removed to achieve the desired effect.

This is one reason why LASIK is far superior to PRK for reducing hyperopia. Indeed, I have never corrected farsightedness with PRK. The protective flap is even more important when treating farsightedness than when correcting nearsightedness. The LASIK flap covers the lasered area, making recovery easier and diminishing regression. Moreover, it is easy to see why a larger flap is necessary for hyperopic corrections. The protective flap must have a large enough diameter to cover the laser trench, which is nearer the outer edge of the cornea than a myopic treatment.

Correction of farsightedness requires the most advanced technology. Doctors must use the new scanning excimer lasers that allow the smoothest ablations and the latest keratome surgical instruments that create a large LASIK flap. The small-beam lasers produce a more blended effect than the older large-beam models. It takes time for the FDA to approve every new mechanical medical device. This is why, initially, U.S. patients had to go to Mexico or Canada to have farsightedness treated surgically with state-of-the-art lasers that were built in the U.S.

AVOIDING H-LASIK COMPLICATIONS

Doctors worry about many of the same rare complications when treating either nearsightedness or farsightedness. Problems are avoided by carefully screening candidates, by using the latest surgical techniques, and by taking advantage of the most advanced scanning lasers. Physicians must use the new keratome surgical instrument that creates the large flap needed to treat hyperopia.

The laser correction has to be perfectly centered so that the patient looks through the correct part of the newly sculpted lens. In other words, the doctor must know exactly how to avoid "decentered" ablations or off-center treatments because a poorly placed laser correction can lead to a drop in the patient's visual acuity with glasses. Imagine that you are creating a "peak" on someone's cornea that must be centered right in front of the-line-of-sight. Looking at the cornea from the side (at its profile), the slope of the curve is steeper for surgically corrected farsighted patients than for nearsighted ones. If the high point of the curve is off-center, either regular or irregular astigmatism can result.

Following H-LASIK, patients lose the magnifying effect of their bubble-like convex glasses. This means that the images falling on their retinas are significantly smaller after surgery. Hence, some people require an adjustment period to get used to their new, more natural vision.

In my opinion, results with hyperopic LASIK probably will never be as good as those with myopic LASIK on a diopter-per-diopter basis. The reason is that in order to steepen the cornea to treat one diopter of farsightedness, the laser must remove much more tissue than to flatten the cornea for one diopter of nearsightedness. Today, the total amount of hyperopia that can be comfortably treated usually is only +4 or +5 diopters.

PERMANENT LENS IMPLANTS FOR HYPEROPIA

Based on a surgical technique first developed in the 1950s, a new operation is under study that implants a tiny permanent lens within the cornea. Such an "additive" technique may prove to be a better option for farsightedness than the current laser "subtractive," or tissue removal, process. During the implant procedure, a surgeon creates a hinged flap of corneal tissue with an automated microkeratome surgical instrument. The doctor then places a small (5-millimeter) soft hydrogel lens on the residual corneal bed and carefully lays the flap over the implant. A relatively safe procedure when performed by an expert, this operation, which is several years away from FDA approval, shows great promise to correct farsightedness. The lens can be removed if problems occur or replaced if the patient's correction changes.

CHAPTER THREE

PRK: A DIARY OF THE ORIGINAL LASER OPERATION

Achieving the best vision possible in the safest,
most conservative manner is the aim.

—Jeffery J. Machat, M.D.
Excimer Laser Refractive Surgery

I'll never forget lying under the excimer laser, the wild pounding of my heart calmed only by a mild sedative. "I am putting more topical anesthetic drops in your eyes, Allison," said Dr. Slade's surgical technician.

Good, I thought, my breastbone aching with fear. At least my eye won't hurt. I was about to undergo photorefractive keratectomy (PRK), the first laser-based operation designed to reduce nearsightedness by optically sculpting the window of the eye (see fig. 9). Having waited thirty minutes while my doctors tested the excimer laser, I was eager to get my out-patient surgery over with.

"It's a 'noninvasive,' surface procedure," my best friend, Carrie, had said. "No scalpels, no incisions, no heat—only lasering," she had reassured me. "The thin, gel-like outer covering of the cornea is removed, but it naturally regenerates every few days." Since she had

had the surgery herself, she talked as an expert. "PRK is an operation that you must go through with 'both eyes wide open,'" she added without smiling.

When I decided to go under the beam, PRK was the only refractive laser operation available to refocus vision. Ophthalmologists weren't doing the new LASIK procedure yet.

"Are you okay, Allison?" my doctor asked, as he typed my refraction or correction, into the computer that would control the laser. The sleek machine was aimed right at my beautiful big baby blue.

"I'm absolutely terrified," I said. He has a kind voice, I thought. He probably thinks I'm his wimpiest patient.

"This will take less than a half-minute, Allison," Dr. Slade reassured me, slipping a specula under my lid to prevent blinking.

I can stand anything for thirty seconds, I thought, trying to forget the scary lid retractors in the movie A Clockwork Orange. He wants to flatten the curvature of my steep central cornea without changing the shape of my eyelid, I thought, remembering the PRK video in Dr. Slade's office. At least, my fear that I would feel claustrophobic was unfounded.

"Don't forget to tell me exactly what you are doing to my eye, doc. I never like to be left in the dark. No pun intended."

"Right now, I am removing the outer covering of your cornea called the epithelium," Dr. Slade said. "It's a thin, protective membrane that usually grows back quickly. The light will become blurred. Do you feel any pressure, Allison?" he asked as he scraped away at the surface of my eye with a blunt, spatula-like instrument.

No, thank God. I felt only a slight rubbing sensation as I watched an impressionistic kaleidoscope of colors. Four thousand dollars had bought me my own private laser light show.

The itching on the tip of my nose was intense. As I started to lift my arm, the surgical technician gently picked up both my hands, holding them away from my face.

"I am about to use the laser to deliver a pre-programmed number of cool pulses of ultraviolet light energy to the surface of your cornea," Dr. Slade said, examining my eye through his microscope.

"Please look at the red fixation light for me, Allison."

"Okay," I replied, staring at the bright glow with all my might.

"Hold it.... Don't move, Allison," Dr. Slade said.

An invisible light beam was etching a new "lens" on my central cornea—right over my line-of-sight. Vaporized corneal collagen smells like burning hair. I tried to count the noisy laser clicks, but they came too fast. In my mind, I imagined my central cornea flattening to a finely resculpted shape. I recalled some colored pictures of images falling directly on the retina once the eye is refocused.

Suddenly, a terrible thought crept into my sedated brain. Could the laser beam make a hole in my eye?

"Can you stop this thing, or is it set on automatic cruise control?" I asked without thinking.

"Please don't talk now," my doctor said. He had instantly deactivated the laser. *"Your job is to hold perfectly still."* His voice was deadly serious. *"When you started talking, I took my foot off the pedal to stop the laser. Your eye is okay. The excimer is so precise that it only removes a quarter of a micron (a quarter of a millionth of a meter) per pulse."*

Not babbling is something that I've never been good at—not even when I'm almost scared speechless. Luckily, since I was mildly nearsighted—only around -2.5 diopters—my treatment was just about finished.

If I had high myopia or severe astigmatism, I couldn't have had PRK. I find it difficult to believe that some people have worse vision than I did. Patients in the higher ranges of myopia have more problems with haze formation and regression of the effect of PRK surgery. I had no astigmatism; at least at age thirty-three, one part of my body was still symmetrical.

"Your left eye is finished, Allison," Dr. Slade said. "It looks good. That wasn't so bad, was it?"

"No, it wasn't," I murmured with a huge sigh. The surgical assistant started putting copious amounts of anesthetic drops in my other eye. The more the better, I thought.

I wanted both eyes done at the same time. I'm a harried reporter. My boss expects me to remember every major news event of the twentieth century. Even though I make a pauper's salary, everyone craves my "glamorous" job. I dared not take off too much time from work.

Once both eyes were lasered, I sat up. A little dazed, I looked around the room. Staring at the silver hair peeking out from under Dr. Slade's green surgical cap, I suddenly realized that I could see. The assistant helped me stand up and led me into an examining room where Dr. Baker was waiting for me. "How do you feel?" he asked.

"I am exhausted, but I feel fine."

"Can you see any better yet?"

"I think I can see," gazing at him in wonder. If only the initial recovery had been half as easy and pain-free as the surgery.

"It's like looking through water," I noted, hoping my vision would improve quickly.

"That's normal," Dr. Baker said, as he carefully inspected my eye with the slit-lamp microscope. "Your eyesight is hazy because the surface of your cornea isn't smooth yet. You should see better after the initial healing period. How quickly you see well isn't indicative of the quality of your final result."

"I want you to go right home, grab something to eat, and go to bed," Dr. Baker said. "You should take it easy for a few days." He put more drops in my eyes. One topical prescription consisted of a combination of antibiotics and steroids called TobraDex. The other drops were an anti-inflammatory drug called Voltaren. Handing me two tiny bottles, he told me to continue to use the drops every four hours when I was awake. The combination antibiotic-steroid drops help

prevent infection and promote healing. Infection risks are greatest during the first few days before the epithelium has completely covered the cornea. The anti-inflammatory drops decrease the discomfort caused by post-surgical swelling.

Instilling more topical anesthetic drops, Dr. Baker slipped disposable therapeutic-bandage contact lenses in my eyes. "The contacts will protect your corneas from the air and help control the pain. Don't remove them because your eye will hurt if you do. If you accidentally lose a contact lens, come in immediately, and I'll replace it. The oral Demerol is for pain, and the Phenergan is for nausea."

Oh great, I thought. I am going to throw up. What if I get it in my eyes?

"My gynecologist gave me Demerol shots after I had abdominal surgery," I said nervously. "That pain-killer didn't work."

"I'll give you another kind of oral narcotic pain medication to use if the Demerol doesn't help you. Here is a sedative to induce sleep. Do you have your post-operative instruction sheet?"

"Yes," I answered, rummaging through my huge purse.

Dr. Baker told me to avoid alcohol, saying that it should never be used with pain medications. PRK and steroids tend to be drying. Alcohol can make the eyes even dryer. I had the surgery because my eyes already were too dry to wear contacts comfortably.

Dr. Baker emphasized that I must keep my eyes well lubricated between the topical prescription applications. He said to close my eyes after using the drops to keep from dislodging the bandage contact lenses. Artificial tears help the contacts float more freely over the cornea.

"I'll see you early tomorrow morning," Dr. Baker said. "Call me if you have any problems."

My sister was my designated driver. I still felt good when I arrived home because the anesthetic drops hadn't worn off yet. But within twenty minutes my enraged eyes started transmitting nasty messages to my brain. I believe in living for the moment, but this was one moment I wanted to exorcise from my life. Each eye had a large corneal abrasion. The windows of my soul hurt—they deeply resented having their protective epithelial coating scraped away. It is not the lasering that inflicts the pain. Most of the second corneal layer called "Bowman's membrane" was gone, leaving my lasered inner cornea unprotected from the air. Unlike the epithelium, Bowman's never grows back. Only a thin bandage contact lens separated each eye from hot soup steam, car exhaust, and my long-haired cat's dander. Obviously, I was one of the unlucky 10 to 20 percent of patients destined to suffer post-operative pain. I marveled how my friend returned to her paperwork four days after her operation.

I swallowed my sedative and Demerol. Within minutes, I was asleep. Five hours later I woke up. Grabbing the phone, I frantically dialed my doctor's emergency number.

"The Demerol isn't working," I said, needing reassurance that my eyes would stop pumping painful probes through my brain. "My left eye only has a mild, deep, dull ache, but the pain in my right eye is excruciating. Both eyes are red, and my lids are puffy. Could I be getting an infection already? I refinanced my car to pay for this misery," I said crossly, my nose running.

"I'm so sorry that you hurt," Dr. Baker said kindly. "It will get better. Since you are only about six-hours post-op, I don't think that you have an infection. Some patients have pain, and some don't. Try the other pain medication, Allison. Ice packs should help. If you want to come to the office, we will be happy to see you."

Within minutes after taking my pills and putting more drops in my eyes, I fell back to sleep. When I woke up the next morning, my eyes felt better, even though they were still scratchy. My sister drove me to the eye clinic. Wearing a wide-brimmed black hat and dark sunglasses, I felt like a hungover movie queen hiding from the blinding light of day.

"*I know you hurt last night. Health-wise, your eye looks good.*" Examining my cornea through the slit-lamp microscope, Dr. Baker said, "*How do you feel?*"

"*I still feel like I have grit in my eyes, but they don't hurt quite as much,*" I said. He is a sweet man, I thought.

"*Your eyes should feel a little better each day,*" my doctor said. "*What is your impression of your vision this morning?*"

"*My vision is pretty amazing. I can see in the distance fairly well, but when I glanced at the morning headlines, my eyes felt strained. When I even think of the scorching white sun, they start tearing. The glare is so bad that I just want to sit in a dark room with sunglasses on.*"

"*Remember that during the healing period, you may be farsighted for a few weeks or even as long as a couple of months. We purposely overcorrect PRK patients a little bit because people usually regress. In other words, you should lose some of the effect of the surgery as you heal. Initially, you may have eye strain, fatigue, or headaches when you do a lot of close work, but using your eyes won't harm them. You also might be sensitive to light at first, but the photophobia will diminish with time. Let's see how well you can read the eye chart.*"

To my absolute delight, I could read the 20/40 line with my left eye and the 20/50 line with right eye, although I still seemed to be looking through water. This is too good to be true, I thought. It was.

"*You are doing great,*" Dr. Baker said. "*Come back to see me in three days, and I'll remove the bandage contact lenses. Don't be alarmed if your vision seems to get a little worse during the initial healing phase. As the epithelium starts to grow back, the surface of the cornea becomes less smooth than when its covering is completely gone. From day four to day seven it is normal for your vision to be worse than at day one. The epithelium usually covers the cornea in about three days, but it is still thinner (only two cells thick) than nor-*

mal. It should build up to about six cells in about one to three months. As the epithelium thickens back to its normal profile, your near vision should improve."

Dr. Baker reminded me to avoid getting shampoo or anything else in my eyes. Of course, I dared not swim for two weeks. No eye makeup for a week. Now everyone would know that my eyebrows and lashes are as blond as my hair. The idea made me slightly uneasy.

"Remember you need 20/40 visual acuity to drive," he said. "It might be a week or two before you can get behind the wheel. Take it slowly. Your depth perception probably has changed."

Driving was the last thing on my mind. I'd planned my operation during my vacation—what a trip!

I first learned about PRK from Carrie, who had sailed right through the surgery and recovery period. She's the one who had said that PRK is "noninvasive." "It was like a miracle!" she told me, speaking with the fervor of the newly converted. She had only mild discomfort for the first four hours after her operation. Carrie said: "It is not as bad as getting a dab of shampoo in your eyes. I only needed a little Advil. Within twenty-four hours, the worst was over." Carrie's optometrist had told her that she was a good candidate for laser surgery because her refractive error was mild. She had little astigmatism, and her eyes weren't dry.

I now understood what Dr. Slade meant when he said that people react to surgery differently. My friend had little post-operative discomfort, but my eyes were uncomfortable for three days, although the pain peaked in the middle of the first night. "The eye can really hurt," my surgeon said. "It is laced with nerves. The therapeutic contact lenses and medications usually alleviate much of the pain, but some people are still uncomfortable during the first night after PRK."

The inflammatory healing response increases with the number of laser pulses and depends on many factors, such as the quality of the laser-beam, the degree of nearsightedness, and the wetness of the cornea. An endless combination of variables interacts with each individual's own wound-healing characteristics and may affect PRK results. Interestingly enough, the severity of discomfort typically has little to do with the degree of correction. Even though the deeper the laser goes—and thus the more variable the healing process—the same amount of surface epithelium (7 millimeters in diameter) is removed whether the patient has a -1 diopter or -4 diopter correction. Hence, the diameter of the painful corneal abrasion is the same no matter what the correction. In addition, people with dry eyes have more pain than patients with a good tear film.

"PRK is real high-tech, science fiction stuff," my friend Carrie had told me. "My vision was 20/25 one week after surgery. It is 20/20 now. Seeing is believing," she added.

Results with PRK are extremely dependent on the range of nearsightedness and on the individual healing response. For mild to moderate myopia, 91.4 percent of PRK patients attain 20/40 or better uncorrected visual acuity, and 63 percent achieve 20/20 or better. Best-corrected vision may be reduced by one to two lines for a few weeks after PRK, but visual acuity with glasses generally recovers by three to four weeks in most patients. In one study, 13 percent of moderately or severely nearsighted PRK patients with greater than -5 diopters of myopia have lost two or more lines of best-corrected visual acuity (vision with new glasses) on the eye chart six months after surgery. So even though PRK has been approved by the FDA for up to -7 diopters of correction using sanctioned lasers, PRK probably should not be the first choice for patients with greater than -5 diopters of myopia or -1.75 diopters of astigmatism. People with higher myopia tend to develop haze and regress after PRK. Some patients have lost some of the effect of the treatment as late as a year or more after surgery.

Subclinical haze, which is collagen protein, usually develops as the inner cornea heals. You can't see most haze with the naked eye.

Viewing the cornea under the magnification of the slit-lamp micro-scope, doctors say that mild haze looks like little pinpoint spots. Such fine haze generally doesn't perceptively interfere with vision, so people can see right through mild haze. Fortunately, it usually diminishes with time. Sometimes these translucent spots form a little matrix-like net that resembles a finger-print on clear glass. If the haze worsens, it can noticeably block the pathway of light.

Some people have such an aggressive wound-healing response after PRK that the haze becomes severe. If it fails to resolve, the cornea can become permanently scarred. Persons with high myopia are the most at risk. If significant haze occurs over the line of sight, patients can lose some effect of the surgery. In other words, they may end up undercorrected with haze and develop side effects such as glare and halos. Even their vision with glasses may worsen. Additional surgery may be necessary not only to remove the haze, but also to treat the residual nearsightedness.

Haze sounded like something I definitely didn't want. My friend had little problems with haze after the first week. "It goes away," she said, explaining that haze formation following PRK for low myopia usually clears with time.

I'm a hopeless optimist. Since I was less nearsighted than Carrie, I discounted the possibility of haze for me.

Dr. Slade told me that doctors are unable to predict exactly how patients will heal after PRK, despite the excimer laser's phenomenal precision. "How you heal will affect your final visual outcome," he explained. "With any operation, complications can occur. Infections have occurred, although they are rare."

Age and sex influence the healing process. Some people are rapid healers and others heal slowly. Older patients have a less robust immune system and a slower healing response than younger people. Patients over age forty have the fewest problems with regression and are the most intolerant of an overcorrection leading to farsightedness.

Young, extremely nearsighted men often are the most aggressive heal-ers. Requiring higher doses of steroid eye drops, these men may have more problems with haze formation, myopic regression, and pain than other patients. A few severely nearsighted people have developed the complication known as "irregular astigmatism," a fine wrinkling of the corneal surface. Another problem is delayed epithelial healing. It is often associated with a loose or tight fitting bandage contact lens or severely dry eyes. Some of these patients have had haze formation. Looking at the eye with the microscope shows that healing continues for at least six to eighteen months.

"Don't worry," Carrie had said. "I had no noticeable complica-tions." Her results were excellent and stable. She was so excited about her new vision that she neglected to mention that she put drops in her eyes for three months. To remember the medication, she had worn the bottle on a string around her neck. Of course, Dr. Baker told me that I would need topical steroids four times a day for three to six months to diminish haze formation and reduce the rate of regression. That didn't sound too bad. Unfortunately, I have never been good at doing anything four times a day, with one exception—I never forget to eat. To remember the drops, I had to set my alarm clock to remind me, but sometimes I forgot to take it or my medicine with me.

Before my surgery, both doctors asked me if I was pregnant. Refractive surgeons usually don't do PRK for a woman who is preg-nant or breast-feeding. Said Dr. Slade: "The steroid eye drops go into the blood stream. We never want to take a chance of affecting a baby. Furthermore, the vision of expectant women can fluctuate, changing the measurements needed for eye surgery. Finally, hormonal fluctua-tions may influence the healing process." He didn't think my birth control pills would be a problem.

Three days later, talking to Dr. Baker, I said, "My vision fluctuates as you said it might. I don't see quite as well as the day after surgery. I guess the epithelium is growing back."

"I think that your vision will improve once your eye settles down," Dr. Baker predicted, removing the bandage contact lenses. *"The epithelium has almost covered the wound."*

It felt great to get rid of the contacts. They helped at first, but now they were becoming uncomfortable.

By the fifth post-surgical day, the antibiotic component of the TobraDex was starting to burn like fire. Dr. Slade changed my medication to steroid drops only, which made my eyes feel much better.

One week later, I was back at the clinic. I had written down a long list of questions: "My vision is still hazy," I complained to Dr. Baker. "When will the halos around the lights at night go away?"

"When I look at your cornea through the slit-lamp microscope, I can see a little mild haze. It is related to the healing process and should get better over time. The halos also should become less prominent. You are faithfully using the eye drops that I gave you, right?"

"Well, most of time," I said, fudging. I didn't want to admit that I had forgotten to use them about half the time.

"Allison, it is vital that you use the steroid eye drops." He said that how I complied with my medication orders would have a key effect on how well I healed. "We have done our part. Now, it is up to you to do yours. We don't want you to lose what you have gained," he added, pointing to the eye chart.

"The letters aren't as black as last week," I said, suddenly overwhelmed with depression. I remembered reading that the epithelium, which is naturally shaped like a concave lens, might grow back thicker in the center than before the surgery, negating some of the effect.

"Your vision is 20/70 in both eyes today," Dr. Baker said.

"Have I already regressed?" I asked, bitterly. This can't be happening to me, I thought, both eyes filling with tears.

"Allison, your epithelium has thinly covered your cornea, but the surface isn't smooth yet. It is ruffled from normal healing. Your vision should gradually get better, but you must faithfully use your eye drops.

The steroids have a stabilizing effect on the cornea. They are extremely important during the wound-healing period."

The steroids affect how the inner cornea remodels itself. A little new collagen forms in the superficial stroma or middle corneal layer. The drops also help keep the epithelium from hypertrophying—growing back too profusely.

"Your epithelium is probably about two cells thick now; in time we want it to return to about six cells—as it was before surgery. We don't want the membrane to build up too much more. In addition, the steroids also reduce haze formation."

"We warn patients not to juggle their medication," Dr. Baker continued. "Some people think that eye drops are like mouthwash. But they are strong medications that enter the blood stream. One lady said the steroids made her eyes feel so good that she doubled the dosage. With PRK, the drops have an important effect on the refractive result. In other words, by medicating herself, she increased the chance of overcorrecting her vision. In addition, the extra steroids elevated her intra-ocular pressure temporarily."

Another week passed. I was already back at work. By this time my near vision was improving—the colors were brighter than before my surgery. I was beginning to see clearly why my friend recommended PRK to me. I was able to do my paper work, but no brain surgery.

At two-and-a-half weeks post-op, I started chasing news stories again. The stress of my hectic job seemed to affect my eyesight. One day, while I was interviewing someone, the huge two-belled alarm in my purse started blaring away. I couldn't remember my eye drops without it. When I put them in, everyone wanted to know all the details of my surgery. Would I recommend PRK? I would let them know in a few months. It was taking longer to get my results than I had hoped. One doesn't just have laser surgery and fly eagle-eyed to Bermuda the next day.

Dr. Baker had to check my eyes monthly while I was using the steroids four times a day. He monitored the pressure within my eyes; nearly 10 percent of patients have increased intra-ocular pressure with long-term steroid use. It also occasionally can lead to "ptosis," or a drooping of the upper eyelid, which usually resolves when the steroids are discontinued. In addition, doctors worry that extended steroid use might accelerate cataract formation. Furthermore, the dosage must be reduced slowly. The risk of haze and scarring of the cornea increases if the steroids are discontinued abruptly.

By the time I was "weaned" off the eye drops at four months after my surgery, my vision was 20/40 with both eyes. Dr. Baker said I still had a tiny bit of haze, but I didn't notice it. He called it subclinical. The halos around the lights at night were less bothersome now. I wore glasses only to drive in dim light. I was starting to take my new eyesight for granted. One gets used to normal really quickly.

Am I pleased with my new vision? Definitely. Have I enthusiastically told all my nearsighted friends about PRK? Well… no, I haven't. I would like to share my good fortune, but I had hoped for quicker results. Longing for better vision, I discounted my doctors' pre-surgical admonition that my final outcome would take time. Unlike my friend Carrie, I'm hesitant to recommend an elective eye operation that might hurt. I remember how angry I was at her the night after my surgery. Maybe such a defensive position is a little selfish, but at least it is safe—no one will be unhappy with me if they have problems.

Allison

CHAPTER FOUR

ARE YOU A CANDIDATE FOR CORRECTIVE SURGERY?

Everything that we behold comes from the unknown.
Our physical body, the physical universe—anything
and everything that we can perceive through our senses—
is the transformation of the unmanifest, unknown,
and invisible into the manifest, known, and visible.

Deepak Chopra
The Seven Laws of Spiritual Success

Am I a candidate? That's one of the first questions most people ask about refractive surgery. What they really want to know is: Will I be happy with my eyesight after my operation? Unfortunately, there is no simple formula to determine answers to these questions. Although general guidelines help eye doctors decide who might benefit from refractive surgery, each candidate must be carefully reviewed on a case-by-case basis. That is why you go to your eye doctor for individualized care and advice. Every operation must be considered in terms of a benefit-to-risk ratio for that specific patient. With elective surgery, it always pays to be conservative.

Figuring out if you might be a good candidate for refractive surgery is as much an art as a science. How will your doctor decide if you will be happy with your outcome? The process is inexact. Looking for people with reasonable expectations, eye doctors try to screen out patients who expect perfect results. Of course, what the laser does is science. With excimer laser surgery, your doctor enters a specific set of numbers into the laser's computer, and the software executes the instructions that control the laser pulses. But how does your doctor decide what numbers should be put in the computer? He must consider how your age will affect your wound-healing response and also must enter data in the computer that will produce a result that will work for your individual eyes and lifestyle. It takes long experience talking with many patients before and after each type of procedure to do this well.

Your doctor will want to know if you are happy with your eyesight with contact lenses. If you are, the physician can attempt to duplicate your prescription with laser surgery. If you are thrilled with your vision with contact lenses that undercorrect your nearsightedness, your doctor can be more conservative in programming your surgical refraction. In other words, by targeting your correction at slightly under 20/20 in the distance, the risk of making you farsighted or overcorrecting you can be diminished. After discussing your personal expectations, your job, and your hobbies—and studying your eye examination and history—your surgeon must pick the exact numbers to put in the computer that, along with your healing response, will determine your future vision. This is the art of vision correction surgery.

Successful eye surgeons want to match your expectations to what they can deliver. Doctors look for indications that patients are highly motivated to improve their vision. Striving to operate on people who will be pleased with their outcomes, ophthalmologists should avoid performing surgery on anyone who expresses major doubts about a procedure. After years of observing patients' reactions to refractive surgery, physicians who specialize in this field start to develop a "sixth sense" about who will be happy with the results. But no matter how long surgeons have performed laser surgery, they continue to learn more from their patients. Such invaluable experience helps doctors identify people who should avoid having these elective procedures.

The range or degree of your refractive error is a key consideration in determining whether you are a good surgery candidate. Your physician will measure your corrected and uncorrected visual acuity. If you are nearsighted, can you read the 20/30 line on the eye chart? Or do you strain to see the big *E* (about 20/400 on some charts)? Generally, the higher the correction, the greater the motivation to have a laser operation. For a severely myopic patient with healthy eyes such as Karen, who can barely count three fingers at a distance of three feet from her eyes, the benefits of LASIK usually greatly outweigh the risks. For a slightly nearsighted person with 20/40 visual acuity, the potential for improvement, of course, is much less, but the medical risks are approximately the same.

LASIK surgery, unlike radial keratotomy (RK—the older, non-laser operation), can improve a wide range of refractive errors, including farsightedness. Nearsighted persons currently can be treated if their refraction is between -1 and -12 diopters—sometimes, depending on the individual case, up to -14 diopters. Although extremely myopic people need help the most, LASIK can leave some of these patients with an unacceptable amount of residual error, meaning that they still will need glasses for distance. So if your correction is greater than -14 diopters, you may want to wait until medical technology has more to offer you. LASIK could improve your vision, but you probably still would have to wear corrective lenses after surgery. (Read chapter 13, "The New Ever-Changing Peripheral

Technology.") As we covered in detail in chapter 2, the thickness of the cornea is a crucial consideration in determining the upper limits of how much myopia doctors can surgically correct for extremely nearsighted people.

Years ago, in doing refractive surgery before the modern LASIK technique was available, doctors often had to tell extremely near-sighted patients, "We're sorry. You're not a candidate. We can only make your vision about 50 percent better."

Some people would respond, "I'll take it! I would like to have thinner glasses. I want to be less helpless without correction." They had reasons for seeking even a partial improvement in their eye-sight. For them, better was better, whether better was perfect or not.

Other patients would say, "Well, if you only can make my eye-sight 50 percent better, why bother having surgery? I would still have to wear glasses even though they would be thinner." For these patients, not having a refractive operation would be the correct choice.

If you are farsighted, ophthalmologists currently can treat up to about +4 or +5 diopters with hyperopic LASIK, although this operation lacks the accuracy of laser surgery for nearsightedness. Unfortunately, if you have greater than +5 diopters or less than +1 diopter of farsightedness, you probably are not a good candidate for this procedure. As previously mentioned, a few patients with presbyopia might benefit by having hyperopic LASIK. By making these patients more nearsighted in their non-dominant eye by about 1.5 diopters, LASIK can improve close vision.

If you have astigmatism, about how much of this refractive error can your surgeon treat with LASIK? At present, we can attempt to correct up to approximately 7 diopters. For people with higher amounts of astigmatism, LASIK can make them better, but they usually will have some residual refractive error left after sur-gery. Doctors now have better software to correct astigmatism than when they first started treating it. Nevertheless, 3 diopters of astigmatism is much more technically difficult to treat than 3 diopters of myopia.

POSSIBLE CONTRA-INDICATIONS TO REFRACTIVE SURGERY

Some health factors might prevent you from having refractive surgery. Your physician will want to learn your medical and ocular history. Some systemic conditions and eye diseases might adversely affect your surgical outcome. Although only a medical book for eye doctors can begin to cover all the reasons not to undergo a refractive eye operation, let your ophthalmologist know if you have any autoimmune diseases such as rheumatoid arthritis or lupus. If you have diabetes and cannot metabolize sugar properly, your physician needs to know this, too. (It might be a good idea to have a blood test for elevated sugar levels before surgery to make certain that you don't have latent or undiagnosed diabetes.) Uncontrolled diabetes can affect surgical results because such patients have fluctuating visual acuity. Persons with controlled diabetes may be able to have successful laser surgery. Women who are pregnant or nursing must inform their doctor, because changes in hormone levels can affect vision, and the eye drops enter the bloodstream.

Before performing a refractive operation, your physician not only will take your medical history, but must also thoroughly examine your eyes. Is your eyeglass prescription fairly stable? Vision correction surgery usually is not recommended for patients who have progressive myopia (rapidly worsening nearsightedness after maturity), "irregular astigmatism" (a fine wrinkling of the cornea that is difficult to treat surgically), corneal scars, "keratoconus" (a cone-shaped deformity and thinning of the cornea causing severe irregular astigmatism), or atrophy of the eye (decrease in the size of the eye caused by a loss of the nerve supply). Let your doctor know if you have had a herpes zoster infection of the ophthalmic nerve or herpes simplex type I (a disease caused by the same virus that leads to cold sores of the mouth). Your physician also needs to know if your eye has been injured in any way or exposed to toxic irritants.

As the art and science of refractive surgery advances, doctors can operate on patients who formerly could not be considered. LASIK has been performed for patients with glaucoma. People with visually significant optic nerve damage, those with late stage glaucoma, or those who have had an operation for glaucoma are not candidates for this procedure. Some people who have had retinal detachments before refractive surgery and others who have had corneal transplants can be successful LASIK patients. Some eye problems have a negligible impact on the results so that a patient can have vision correction surgery, but each case is unique and requires careful attention to every medical detail.

Should someone with only one healthy eye consider vision correction surgery? Even though LASIK is a safe and effective procedure, the stakes are much higher for this individual. A few surgeons will operate on a patient's only good eye if surgery can help overcome a severe handicap. The person may be risking everything, but she may have everything to gain. Such an individual is taking additional risks, but if having refractive surgery is extremely important to her, it can be an option. Her doctor must thoroughly explain all the risks so that she can carefully weigh them and make an informed decision.

Doctors, of course, do everything humanly possible to reduce the risks for such patients. In some cases, if a person has one healthy eye, and the other one is nearsighted, the ophthalmologist might perform LASIK on the eye with low vision first to see how well the operation works before doing refractive surgery on the good eye. Operating on the weak one first gives the patient and the surgeon at least an opportunity to learn how the person heals. Then, together they could make a more informed judgment on whether to treat the second eye. A doctor who encounters any problems surgically focusing the eye with low vision should avoid operating on the patient's healthy eye.

Oliver, an extremely nearsighted fifty-seven-year-old attorney, could wear his gas-permeable contact lenses, but they were rather uncomfortable. He wondered whether LASIK might be an option if he eventually could no longer wear his lenses. A brilliant mathematician and actuary, Oliver was president of a large publicly traded company, managing a multi-billion-dollar stock portfolio. He spent most of his time looking at numbers on computer screens and financial statements.

Oliver was an extremely stoic patient who seldom complained about anything. "I feel very lucky to see as well as I do," he said. "I have had lots of problems with my eyes. Following a severe herpes simplex Type I infection, I had to have a corneal transplant on my right eye. Then a couple of years later, I had surgery on both eyes for retinal detachments. I don't even own a pair of glasses. Years ago, I had some, but I couldn't see anything with them. I am totally dependent on my contacts, and I am worried because they bother me more every day. Even though I have a -18 diopter correction, my lenses correct me to 20/25 in my dominant eye and 20/50 in my non-dominant one. Can I have LASIK if my contacts eventually become unbearable?"

We have many patients who have had good results with LASIK after having a corneal transplant. We also have patients who have had a repaired detached retina and then had a successful LASIK procedure. Nevertheless, since Oliver can still see with his contact lenses, we advised him to continue wearing them for as long as possible. Although LASIK can theoretically correct his degree of nearsightedness, practically speaking, Oliver is too nearsighted to have excimer laser surgery. Since he has had so many problems with his eyes, he must be carefully watched by an ophthalmologist.

Approaching sixty, Oliver also has the beginnings of cataracts— a generally progressive clouding of the crystalline lenses inside the eyes. As he ages, these lenses will become increasingly cloudy because of further cataract formation. When his cataracts become so dense that his eyesight is poor even with contacts, the cataracts can be removed and each crystalline lens replaced with an artificial one. Such intra-ocular lenses eliminate or diminish nearsightedness, although corrective lenses are necessary to focus close objects. Oliver may be able to avoid cataract surgery for years. Nonetheless, he should not wait until his cataracts become so hard that they are difficult to remove, especially since he has had retinal problems.

Even though many people all over the world have had excellent results with refractive surgery, you might not be a good candidate for these procedures. Here are some reasons why:

- You are happy with your glasses.
- You are pleased with your contact lenses.
- You demand perfect vision or guaranteed results.
- You don't want to accept the risk of eye surgery.
- You have an overwhelming fear of an eye operation.

No matter what your decision, you should make it based on a thorough understanding of the specific procedure that you are considering.

CAN LASER SURGERY HELP AMBLYOPIA (LOSS OF VISION) ASSOCIATED WITH A "LAZY EYE"?

You learn to see. Your vision evolved because as a newborn you opened your eyes and looked at the fascinating world around you.

During the early months of your life, your vision improved. Soon, you attained the ability to use your two eyes together. No one is born with this skill. If you had been deprived of light stimulation during your first few years, your adult brain would not know how to see. Without sight-giving light, the normal neurological connections fail to grow properly. Your eyes need the early stimulation of a clear image to develop the retinal cells that send the proper impulses to your brain. To keep from losing your precious sense of sight, you must continue to use your eyes. Even if no ophthalmic disease process is present, if you stop using one eye to its capacity, over time it can develop "amblyopia" or a loss of visual acuity. Wanting to see clearly, the brain suppresses the weaker image if there is too much disparity between the two eyes.

Can refractive surgery improve your eyesight if you suffer from amblyopia? LASIK may help some adults with this condition see better, but the laser cannot cure a loss of the brain's ability to see. If you have a refractive error in either or both eyes, refractive surgery should put them more in focus. Ophthalmologists can surgically reduce the nearsightedness, farsightedness, or astigmatism so that a clear image falls on the retina. We are unable, however, to repair the way the retinal cells send images to the brain. If you have a large difference in the refractive power of your eyes, putting them more in focus will help balance your vision. For example, if you have -6 diopters of moderate nearsightedness in your amblyopic eye and -1 diopter in your best eye, LASIK might reduce the myopia in both eyes to under -1 diopter. Nevertheless, even if the refractive error in each eye is largely eliminated, the vision with the amblyopic eye will still be below par. Sadly, some people with amblyopia have no benefit from being more in focus. If they cannot see because of a tilting of the retinal cells, LASIK cannot help. Refractive surgery is unable to make the eye's vision better than its maximum potential.

What Causes Amblyopia?

Most causes of amblyopia are related to disuse of the eye. The two most common are a direct result of an imbalance between the two eyes—either muscular or focusing. Both can lead to the suppression of the vision of the weaker eye. If you look through only one eye, the ignored eye over time can lose some of its ability to see.

Normally, our eyes work in unison. Moving together, they target an object, fusing its image. But if the muscles that move the eye are uncoordinated, all the benefits of binocular vision with both eyes focused on the same object are lost. A muscle weakness can cause the eye to be misaligned, leading to a condition called "strabismus" by doctors. About half of the children with this problem ignore the image from the deviating eye. Left untreated, the "lazy" eye can lose vision.

Doctors also look for an imbalance in the focusing power of the eyes. Called "anisometropia," a large unnoticed difference in the refractive error between the eyes can cause amblyopia. If one of a child's eyes is more nearsighted, farsighted, or astigmatic than the other one, the eye with the most blurred image turns off. The youngster may be unaware that one eye isn't functioning properly. Unless the eye crosses, it usually looks normal. Farsightedness may cause the eyes to cross because of the intense focusing effort of the crystalline lens. In addition, a large uncorrected out-of-focus condition can eventually result in loss of vision. In other words, extreme nearsightedness, astigmatism, or farsightedness can cause amblyopia if the refractive error isn't optically or surgically corrected.

Any serious opacity that interrupts the path of light through the eye to the brain of a child can cause amblyopia if left untreated. If a youngster with perfectly healthy eyes wears a patch over the same eye for an extended period, after about the age of seven, the vision in the unused eye will never be normal. Years ago, people inaccurately thought that a condition they called "postmarital amblyopia" was caused by sexual excess.

When most people think of amblyopia they recall a child with a lazy or "crossed" eye. The youngster may have poor eyesight through the wayward eye. It probably turned because it had a much greater refractive error than the straight eye or because of muscle weakness. Biofeedback keeps our eyes straight; if one begins to turn, we see double. To avoid seeing two images, the child's brain turns off the weak eye. All the muscles that control the amblyopic eye relax, leaving it to "float" to its rest position—which might be turned in, up, down, or out. If the wayward eye lacks the acuity capabilities of the other eye, over time the brain will suppress the poorer image. In this way, a child avoids "diplopia," or seeing two images of unequal clarity. Trained to receive images from both eyes, the adult brain may see double if the person develops strabismus.

Amblyopia affects about 4 percent of the population, but the condition can be corrected if diagnosed and treated during a child's early years. To bring the eyes more into alignment, the youngster may wear a corrective eye patch over the best eye to force the weak eye to work. Depending on the case, the ophthalmologist also may recommend injections that temporarily relax an opposing eye muscle or surgery to reposition some of the eye muscles.

MANAGING THE FEAR OF EYE SURGERY

Most people who need corrective lenses are absolutely fascinated with the idea of improving their eyesight, but they fear an eye operation. All of us instinctively realize that sight is our most precious sense. After performing thousands of LASIK procedures, I believe that patient education is the key to managing the fear of eye surgery. Unfortunately, some patients handle this anxiety by hastily scheduling the procedure before they have time to think about it. In fact, it is much better to educate oneself thoroughly first. Patients need to be knowledgeable about the specific operation they are contemplating. They deserve a detailed understanding of how a procedure might benefit them and of how it might fall short of their expectations.

There is never a reason to rush into a refractive operation. LASIK is elective surgery—people can continue to wear their glasses or contacts. Unlike heart or cancer surgery, which is crisis management medicine, near- and farsighted patients have no pressure to have their eyes surgically refracted. Personal control over a decision-making process sometimes diminishes anxiety. Over time, many people can eventually work through much of their fear of eye surgery. They can thoroughly examine the various treatment choices to decide if an operation has the potential to help. They have the option of having vision correction surgery next month, next year, or never.

By studying the LASIK procedure, you will learn that your apprehension is largely unnecessary. LASIK is a reasonably safe operation *in expert hands,* although no one can guarantee perfect results. Even though doctors always worry about possible infection with any surgery, the risk is extremely small with LASIK. In fact, this technique has now advanced to the point where you probably have less chance of getting an eye infection from having LASIK one time than from wearing contact lenses on a continuing basis. After LASIK, the eye heals almost to its original state. If you get hit in the eye after the LASIK healing period, your eye's "burst" strength will be as strong as before surgery. Furthermore, the chances that LASIK will damage your eye are slight. Nevertheless, as mentioned earlier, rare complications can occur, and some can be permanent. If a problem does arise after surgery, it usually happens during the first day or two following treatment.

Unfortunately, even contact lenses are not totally safe. Problems associated with wearing them have been discussed in the *New England Journal of Medicine*. According to a Sept. 21, 1989, article, the most serious adverse effect of wearing contact lenses is "ulcerative keratitis," an ulceration of the corneal epithelium with an underlying inflammation of the corneal stroma. Although rare, this condition—which can be associated with a permanent loss of vision—can develop with soft, hard, and rigid gas-permeable contact lenses.

The risk of corneal ulceration increases significantly when patients wear extended-wear lenses while *sleeping*. A study at six major eye centers around the country found that 62 percent of those using extended-wear lenses and 11 percent of those using daily-wear lenses wore them overnight, at least occasionally. The authors write: "Rough estimates of incidence that take overnight use into account can be obtained if one disregards differences in geography and time between the two studies and combining their results: the estimated incidences are 2 to 3 per 10,000 for daily-wear lenses worn on a strict daily-wear basis, and 22 to 32 per 10,000 for extended-wear lenses worn overnight." Although the refractive, optical, and cosmetic benefits of contacts are well-known, their overnight use is questionable.

Once you understand the LASIK procedure, including the creation of the protective flap and the submicron precision of the excimer laser, you will look upon this operation more as refractive surgeons do. Ophthalmologists have more than fifty years experience operating within the inner layers of the cornea. At this writing, we have over a ten-year history of using the excimer laser on people. Once the hinged flap—which has natural adhesive properties—is repositioned properly, it heals almost to its original state. The cornea's liquid nutritional supply is sucked through the tissue from front to back. The flap adheres to the corneal bed at several levels; it rapidly reattaches itself at the top two layers. Over time, some fibers of the middle layer of the cornea, which is 80 percent water, cross-link. Since the cool excimer laser focuses vision by reshaping the front of the eye, or inner cornea—as opposed to going deep inside the eye—the eye's interior structures remain untouched. Consequently, some medical risks are reduced. Even if a patient were in a devastating automobile accident, and the flap were ripped loose, the person would still be able to see fairly well, although someone who was severely myopic before surgery might need a tissue graft. In an extremely rare emergency, the cornea, unlike the retina and optic nerve at the back of the eyeball, usually can be successfully replaced. (See chapter 11 for a detailed discussion of corneal transplants.)

What patients worry about most is that they might lose some or all of their vision. Extremely nearsighted people are especially concerned because they are acutely aware of how poor eyesight affects every phase of life. Since the chances that someone will lose vision with LASIK are remote, a "failure" usually means that the patient's visual acuity did not improve enough to make the person happy with the result. All things considered, the most valid criticism of LASIK is that, even though eyesight without glasses improves, some people still need correction after surgery.

One of the most effective ways to alleviate some fear of eye surgery is to obtain enough background information to develop confidence that your surgeon is highly skilled and experienced in all types of refractive procedures, but especially in the operation you are considering. You may wish to observe a procedure on your doctor's TV monitor. At some clinics, you can watch surgery through a glass window. Others have videotapes or CD-ROMs showing each type of procedure.

We recommend that you talk with several of your doctor's patients—those near your age and range of vision who have had the procedure you are contemplating. Since LASIK is a quick out-patient operation, discussing it with others usually proves reassuring. Many surgery patients will enthusiastically tell you about all the wonderful benefits of improved vision. Talking with them should lessen the fear of pain that keeps many people from having corrective eye surgery. Even though everyone is different, following such a person through the entire operation can help you see what it is like to undergo this procedure. Most LASIK patients lay down under the laser, have the surgery, get up, and walk out the door, amazed that they can see better immediately.

Mary, a thirty-five-year-old flight attendant, overcame much of her fear by talking with her prospective doctor's patients:

> The surgeon could see that I was terrified of having any operation on my eyes. He suggested that I talk with a few of his LASIK patients, including those who required a second operation. This seemed like a good idea, but I wanted to pick the patient. I didn't want to talk with someone he did four years ago. I said: "I want to actually follow a patient through the LASIK procedure—from start to finish."
>
> "Good idea," he replied. "I do LASIK every Thursday and Friday. Come in when you have time."
>
> Early the next morning, I started talking with people in the reception area who were scheduled to have LASIK that day. I met a friendly forty-year-old accountant from Detroit named Peter. He was almost as nearsighted as I was. Peter said his brother had LASIK surgery six months earlier.
>
> "Eric, that's my brother," Peter said, "was pleased with his results. I hope I do as well," he added, appearing very nervous.
>
> "My sister is an optometrist," Peter's wife said. "She sometimes refers patients to laser surgeons. Since optometrists don't operate, they should have no vested interest in persuading you to have eye

surgery. A trusted optometrist often can give you an educated, non-biased opinion. I would check with several, however. Some are much more knowledgeable about refractive surgery than others."

I watched Peter's operation through a glass window. The entire procedure for both eyes took only fifteen minutes. His eyes were anesthetized, and he certainly didn't appear to have any pain. Afterward, he seemed to recover immediately. He got up and walked through the reception area. He had no black patches on his eyes—not even clear plastic shields. He wasn't crying or anything. On the contrary, he was smiling.

When Peter saw his wife, he said, "Honey, I can see! It is unbelievable." He looked so happy. He not only embraced his wife, he hugged everybody—both doctors, the assistants, and even me. About a month later, I called Peter in Detroit. He was still pleased with his new eyesight. He wore glasses only to drive at night.

Most patients feel more comfortable about having LASIK when they realize that it is the vision correction surgery that most eye doctors prefer to have on their own eyes. Nowadays, more ophthalmologists and optometrists are asking me to do this procedure for them. Since they are often my friends of long-standing, these surgeries are not totally stress-free for me. Although eye doctors are highly knowledgeable patients who are keenly aware of the advantages and limitations of refractive surgery, the demands of their job leave no tolerance for poor vision.

In 1997, Stephen F. Brint, M.D., my good friend of over ten years, asked me to perform LASIK on both of his eyes. A well-known refractive and cataract surgeon, Steve works on a tight schedule—he wanted to squeeze in his LASIK procedure in Houston between a working trip in Europe and a Fourth of July holiday weekend in Aspen. He hoped to see well enough to operate on patients right after his vacation.

The day of his LASIK operation, Steve, who is a clinical professor of ophthalmology at Tulane University in New Orleans, arrived at my office with an entourage of seven or eight people, including a film crew to produce a video of his surgery for his patients. He seemed totally laid back—not frightened at all.

One week earlier, Steve, Dr. Baker, and I had discussed his case at length while we were attending the International Society of Refractive Surgery meeting in Florida. Behaving like a patient rather than a doctor, Steve asked our opinion about questions that he has answered hundreds of time for his own patients. A down-to-earth guy, Steve knows that when a doctor treats himself as a patient, he is neither a good patient nor a good doctor. Together, the three of us carefully studied the topographic maps showing the "hills and valleys" of his cornea. Like all patients, Steve asked what we thought his vision would be like after surgery. I asked him whether he was pleased with his pre-surgical correction with his old glasses, which wasn't very good. He simply said, "Sure." Since they failed to correct all of the astigmatism in his right eye, I felt that I had a good chance to make him exceedingly happy.

During his pre-op examination in Houston, Dr. Baker and I refracted Steve twelve times each to determine his exact correction before we set up his surgical plan. Steve was completely willing to submit himself to our routine, but he finally said: "Whatever you decide is fine, but I think that's close enough. Let's use *that* number." Every single refraction was videotaped. In fact, each part of Steve's case was documented on videotape.

Right before Steve's surgery, several people asked me whether I was nervous. "Yes," I admitted, noting that my stress had not yet reached the level of a few years ago when I operated on my mom and dad. I removed their cataracts. When working under unusual conditions, I avoid errors by following a routine intra-operative plan. No matter how well I know the patient, I never fail to ask him to spell his name so that I can double-check it with the chart as I enter the refraction into the laser's computer. My surgical assistants always recheck my figures. The more distractions in the operating room, the greater the importance of such standardized systems and procedures.

Steve's surgery went well. He could see much better immediately following LASIK. Although at first he felt like he was looking through a foggy windshield, the mist lifted after four or five hours. Later, when Steve looked through the operating microscope, he was extremely relieved that he could see the surgical field clearly. Later, only three days after his operation, his vision was clear enough to perform thirty cataract operations with the microscope. About one week post-op, his uncorrected visual acuity was 20/30 in his left eye and 20/25 in his right eye, the one with significant pre-surgical astigmatism. Two months after LASIK, he said that his unaided vision was as good as or better than when he wore soft contact lenses. He was glad to be free of the worry that a contact lens might pop out of his eye. It was a special honor to be Steve's surgeon, but my greatest reward was that he was pleased with his results.

Since LASIK is a rather new procedure, a knowledge of how it evolved can alleviate some of the fear that surrounds eye operations. As illustrated by the fascinating history of refractive surgery covered later in this book, eye doctors have learned a great deal over many years about how to correct vision surgically. They have an in-depth understanding of the eye's healing process, and they now have advanced precision instruments with which to operate. Nevertheless, even for some informed people, the fear of any eye surgery is insurmountable.

Several years ago, a nearsighted patient from Italy named Paul came to our office. Considering him an excellent LASIK candidate, his ophthalmologist had sent us his records. After his eye examination, Paul said that he wanted to have the procedure. Then he read the long, legally binding, informed-consent form.

"Well," he said, "this says that there's a chance that I can go blind from this surgery."

"That is true," I replied. "If the procedure is done improperly, you could permanently lose all or part of your vision. The chance of infection—which we can usually cure—is very low, and the risk of blindness is extremely remote."

"Well, why would I want to have any surgery that could make me blind?" asked Paul.

"I understand your point," I said. "But with any surgery, there is always a chance that something could go wrong."

Paul returned to Italy without having refractive surgery. He had overcome his fear of flying but not his anxiety about having an operation on his eyes.

Eye doctors—who see blind patients on a daily basis—are probably more terrified of losing vision than anyone. Although your surgeon can explain all the risks and rewards of refractive surgery, if he says to you, "You could lose your vision," how can you, as a sighted person, possibly understand what such a loss would mean?

A few years ago, a Continental Airlines DC-10 pilot named Jim—whose job required 20/20 distance vision *with* corrective lenses—asked me to perform LASIK on his eyes. The big question was: Could he pass the FAA flight physical after LASIK? I believed that he had a good chance of passing the eye test because before surgery his glasses corrected him to 20/15, which is better than normal. Even if Jim had lost a slight amount of best-corrected visual acuity (BCVA) after LASIK—which seldom happens in expert hands—he still probably could be refracted with glasses to 20/20. Not everyone has an optical system capable of perfect eyesight even with correction. If Jim's pre-surgical vision had been barely 20/20, I would have hesitated to operate on him because—if he had lost any BCVA—he not only would have failed his vision test but he would have lost his job.

Another important factor in our favor was the reduction of the minification effect that occurs following refractive surgery. Since Jim's pre-surgical vision was -7 diopters, we knew that he would gain about one line on the eye chart because he would no longer wear thick-edged glasses. If LASIK corrects a patient to 20/20 without lenses, this reduction in the minification effect sometimes can improve his visual acuity to 20/15 with contacts or glasses. After surgery, Jim's final vision was 20/20 with glasses and 20/25 without them, which means that he only wears glasses to fly a plane. Since Jim is a pilot, he is accustomed to managing risk. He was willing to put his job on the line to have refractive surgery. Even though he thoroughly understood the downside, he felt comfortable that the odds were in his favor.

Chapter Five

Are Your Expectations Realistic?

Success is defined as meeting patient expectations
rather than a visual goal.

—Jeffery J. Machat, M.D.

The key to success for any elective procedure is meeting patients' expectations. Using state-of-the-art refractive technology, can your doctor match your surgical outcome to your goals? If you are considering vision correction surgery, it is essential that you gain a realistic picture of what these procedures might offer you. As you now know, the modern LASIK technique probably can greatly improve your unaided vision, but no operation can promise perfect results. Most people want perfect 20/20 unaided visual acuity, but they will be satisfied with 20/25 or 20/30 uncorrected vision. LASIK gives mildly and moderately nearsighted patients an over 90 percent chance of driving during the day without glasses. Some refractive surgery patients, however, still need glasses to see well in low-light conditions such as looking at exhibits in a poorly lit museum or driving at night.

No matter how nearsighted or farsighted you are before surgery, afterward you may want a second operation if you are left with -1 diopter or more of residual nearsightedness. The last diopter of myopic correction will improve your focus from one meter to infinity. Hence, if you are one diopter undercorrected, you will see clearly up to one meter when you want to be focused not only close up but also in the distance. If LASIK improves your eyesight by several diopters, you will gain lines on the eye chart. Even if your visual acuity isn't 20/20 when viewing a distant object, your vision should improve all the way out to infinity.

Why are some people happy after a refractive operation while others aren't? Basically, two reasons: first is the degree of improvement in their uncorrected vision after surgery. If their eyesight improved from a severe correction of -10 diopters to a mild one of -1 diopter, they probably will be thrilled. If it went from -2 to -0.5 diopters, yes, their vision is better, but they haven't experienced such a dramatic change. Second, what is their reference point—their pre-operative corrected vision? After surgery, people usually compare their post-surgical eyesight without corrective lenses to their best-corrected visual acuity (BCVA) *with* corrective lenses before surgery. For example, if you are corrected from 20/80 to 20/20 with contacts and become 20/30 without them after LASIK, you probably will compare your new 20/30 *uncorrected* vision to your former 20/20 BCVA with your lenses—even though your glasses or contacts still refract you to 20/20 after surgery. You quickly forget that your unaided visual acuity was 20/80 before LASIK.

Most persons with rigid, gas-permeable contact lenses enjoy extraordinarily sharp eyesight. Wearing a perfectly smooth, hard-milled surface on their eyes, some of these patients see better than 20/20, reading the 20/10 or 20/15 line on the eye chart. If they have LASIK, and become 20/20, 20/25, 20/40 or worse without contacts, their new *unaided* vision will lack the crispness possible with gas-permeable lenses. So, after surgery, some of these patients say, "Yes, I can see a lot better now without my contacts, but my vision isn't as sharp as with my gas-perm lenses."

To give patients an idea of what their vision might be like after an operation, we sometimes have them try soft lenses that slightly undercorrect their vision. Nearsighted gas-perm wearers who are unhappy with their eyesight when they try soft contacts may be difficult to please with refractive surgery. People often wear gas-perm lenses because they have significant astigmatism. Non-toric *soft* lenses fail to correct astigmatism. As mentioned earlier, laser operations can reduce astigmatism, but don't always eliminate it. Of course, patients who comfortably wore gas-perm lenses before surgery usually can wear them after LASIK to correct any residual myopia, hyperopia, or astigmatism. In practice, however, people rarely ask for gas-perm lenses after a refractive procedure. Most patients say they aren't worth the trouble.

One happy LASIK patient, who had excellent results, wanted her nearsighted son to have the procedure. A twenty-two-year-old physics student at the University of Houston, he was happy with his gas-permeable contact lenses, which corrected his vision from -5 diopters to 20/15, or better than normal. He had no glasses. Saying that he passes out during any medical procedure, he was not eager to have refractive surgery. It was obvious that he had made an appointment with us to please his mother. Since he was totally unmotivated to have LASIK and since he had excellent, reasonably comfortable vision with his gas-perm lenses, we didn't consider him a good candidate for eye surgery—even though his mother was willing to pay for it. Later, if his rigid contact lenses start bothering him, soft contacts or LASIK still could be an option.

So your correction before surgery will greatly influence how pleased you are with your results. Your eye doctor will carefully consider your current corrective lenses when he begins the difficult job of predicting how happy you'll be after surgery. Wearers of soft contact lenses are probably better LASIK candidates than those with gas-permeable lenses. Surgery patients who have tried both soft and rigid contacts sometimes say their unaided vision after LASIK resembles their former correction with soft contacts rather than their refraction with rigid lenses. Since the latter provide such super sharp eyesight, people wearing these contacts are usually less happy after surgery than soft-lens wearers—even if both groups have the identical post-surgical results.

For extremely nearsighted people looking through the center of thick-edged glasses—especially if they cannot wear contact lenses—LASIK can be a life-changing experience. Their vision should improve dramatically, even though the higher the refractive error the more difficult it is to correct. Such a patient—who may see better after LASIK without glasses than she did before surgery with them—often is easier to please than a mildly nearsighted person whose vision improves slightly after surgery, even though both may end up with similar uncorrected vision. Interestingly enough, a few extremely nearsighted people who have never worn any correction except thick-edged glasses may take a little time to adjust to excellent natural vision. Of course, some highly myopic patients still have to wear thin glasses or contacts after surgery. These folks often say, however, that their vision with their new thin spectacles is much better than with their old thick-edged glasses. Thinner contacts are also easier to wear than thicker ones.

Now, if your soft lenses comfortably provide you with 20/20 visual acuity, should you have LASIK? Our advice is that you carefully consider whether you would be satisfied with your refractive surgery results. Even though many nearsighted LASIK patients achieve 20/20 visual acuity, what if your post-surgical distance vision is, say, 20/30, 20/40, 20/50, or worse without corrective lenses after surgery? Your physician can show you what 20/40 and other refractions are like as you look at the eye chart through dial-up lenses with varying amounts of correction. We recommend that you try living with 20/40 vision before surgery by wearing soft contact lenses that undercorrect you. In Texas, for example, you will need 20/40 visual acuity or better in your worst eye to pass the eye test to drive. Some people can function with such undercorrected eyesight; others demand more precise vision and wear correction after a refractive operation at least part of the time. Even if they still have a slight amount of residual error, they can wear contacts or thin glasses to refine their vision after LASIK. A few patients ask for a repeat operation to try to fine-tune their vision.

Jeanne, a bright-eyed, fifty-year-old librarian, was unable to wear her gas-permeable contacts with comfort. She tried toric soft lenses to correct her -4 diopters of nearsightedness and moderate astigmatism, but they were extremely uncomfortable. Eventually, she was forced to switch to disposable soft contacts. Since Jeanne had astigmatism, her vision was blurry at every distance with these lenses. An avid reader, she wore bifocals over her contacts to correct her presbyopia and astigmatism. Jeanne had a total hysterectomy at age forty-four and had wide emotional swings, even though she took hormone replacement therapy. She complained of allergies, dry eyes, and thinning hair. She had been treated for two eye infections associated with wearing contact lenses. Eager to improve her eyesight, Jeanne had saved her money for two years for refractive surgery.

After talking with Jeanne we believed that LASIK could meet her expectations. She said: "My mom has rheumatoid arthritis. The doctors can do little to help her. There are so many things in life that we have to accept the way they are—that we cannot change. This is one thing that modern medicine can now make better. I'd like to have 20/20 vision without correction, but I'll be happy just to see better without contacts."

After thoroughly examining her eyes and discussing her visual goals, we concluded that Jeanne was a good candidate for refractive surgery. One month after her operation, her vision was 20/30 with both eyes. LASIK decreased her astigmatism from -2.25 diopters to -0.5 diopters, which was extremely mild. Jeanne now seldom wears glasses except to drive or to watch a movie. Able to read without correction most of the time, she only needs magnifiers to see fine print. She had realistic expectations about what refractive surgery could do for her and is overjoyed with her results.

Jeanne said, "My eyes feel more comfortable. They are less red and allergy prone. My vision is much more natural and stable. When I wore contacts, I built up enzyme deposits on them, so my eyesight varied. Of course, I never get contact lens-induced eye infections anymore. I don't actually see better now than I did with my contacts, but my vision seems more consistent."

Refractive surgery patients sometimes need an enhancement or refinement procedure, which always involves significantly more risk than the first operation. Nevertheless, many patients have fine-tuned their vision further with a second LASIK operation. If Jeanne's unaided visual acuity after her first procedure had been undercorrected by -1 diopter or worse, she might have requested additional surgery to try to bring her vision closer to 20/20. (See chapters 11 and 12 for detailed information on enhancement surgery.)

Farsighted LASIK candidates often become our happiest refractive surgery patients. Hyperopia is extremely frustrating, especially as people age. As mentioned earlier, when patients with this refractive error lose their ability to accommodate around age forty, they not only are unable to focus up close, but eventually they cannot see well in the distance. Even if vision correction surgery only corrects them from +4 diopters to +1 diopter, they usually are pleased with their surgical outcome.

Doctors have to be exceedingly careful to avoid surgically over-correcting nearsighted patients to the point that they become far-sighted. As people get older they are less able to tolerate even a slight amount of hyperopia. As they become unable to accommodate or "see through" farsightedness, myopic patients who are over-corrected after refractive surgery are extremely unhappy. Although an overcorrection now can be treated with additional surgery, ophthalmologists purposely slightly undercorrect nearsighted patients to avoid making them farsighted.

Anecdotal stories that circulate among refractive surgeons suggest what type of person might have realistic expectations about refractive surgery. Clinicians with years of experience treating refractive errors surgically say that even the most demanding doctors and attorneys are often better refractive surgery candidates than engineers and architects. Engineers and architects are less accustomed to dealing with the imprecise—they expect all their buildings to be vertical. Since the practice of medicine is a hands-on art form, physicians are used to dealing with results that are less than perfect. In addition, doctors as well as lawyers are all too familiar with risk. Plastic surgeons especially understand that surgery can greatly improve part of the human body, but that results vary considerably from one person to another. Their patients also often make good refractive surgery candidates because their experience with cosmetic surgery has lowered their expectations slightly.

Excellent vision is much more than being able to read the 20/20 line on the eye chart. This is only one measurement of the complex physiological process of sight. You have 20/20 vision, but what's your contrast sensitivity? What's your depth of field? What's your field of vision? How well do you use both of your eyes together? What's your night vision? What's your color vision?

Some people have such poor contrast sensitivity that they fail to discern many different shades of gray. Others cannot see clearly from near to far. Some have a narrow field of vision. If patients' eyes fail to move together, if they cannot see in dim light, or if they are unable to tell red from green, they are still visually impaired, even if their eyes are focused properly.

Some people have 20/20 vision, but they have glaucoma. They see the world through two tiny tunnels. Some folks lack stereo vision; others have double vision. In other words, yes, they can read the 20/20 line on the eye chart, but the quality of their eyesight is poor. Hence, patients can have 20/20 vision as measured by the eye chart and be tremendously unhappy with their vision. If, after surgery, they have residual astigmatism or poor night vision, the quality of their eyesight may be inadequate without glasses. Before surgery, it is your doctor's job to help you consider all the elements of vision as they apply to your eyes.

There also is a profound psychological aspect to testing vision that goes far beyond the ability to function visually. Sometimes patients with 20/20 vision will ask: "What is my vision today?"

We will say: "Well, you're living it. Are you happy?"

Some people reply: "No! No! I want to know if my vision is 20/20 on the eye chart." If we answer: "You just read the 20/20 line," they will say, "Oh, wow! That's great."

But if we joke with them and say, "You're 20/40 today," they say, "Oh...." and look profoundly disappointed. It is almost like patients are asking: Am I normal? Am I okay? Or am I still behind the rest of the population?

CHAPTER SIX

CHOOSING YOUR
REFRACTIVE
SURGEON

*In a profound and mysterious alchemy, sight combines
with memory to energize the will.*
— "The Sense of Sight," *National Geographic*

The onus of finding correct medical care falls largely on the shoulders of the consumer. Nowhere is this more apparent than in the field of vision correction surgery. If you are considering one of these operations, the choice of your eye doctor is absolutely vital to your future vision. Picking an excellent surgeon is probably one of the most critical decisions that you will make about your eyes. You might begin the search by asking your regular eye doctor to identify the leaders in the field. There are national laser centers, some are mentioned in the back of this book, that represent eye doctors throughout the United States and Canada. We recommend that you talk with several experts. Ask who treats the complications that occasionally occur during a refractive operation. It obviously takes more skill to make surgical repairs than to perform a primary operation.

Your eye doctor should be willing to sit down with you, put you at ease, and thoroughly answer all your questions. You will want to know her education and experience. Is your ophthalmologist comfortable doing all types of refractive surgery—including RK, PRK, and LASIK? Ask for her statistical results for the operation you are considering. What percentage of her patients have 20/20 vision after this procedure? What percentage have 20/25, 20/30, 20/40, or worse? Ask if she has researched and published articles in ophthalmology journals on any of these operations. Does she have specialty training in corneal surgery? In other words, is she an expert at operating within the cornea's inner layers? Non-corneal surgeons can do uncomplicated techniques, but corneal surgeons may have an advantage when complications arise.

If you are interested in LASIK, ask your doctor specifically how many of these surgeries she has done and how long she has been doing them. An ophthalmologist who has performed twenty thousand RKs isn't *necessarily* skilled at performing LASIK. Prospective LASIK surgeons must take a special course in this technique, and they must complete a proctored, hands-on training program. Such courses, which manufacturers of the surgical equipment require, qualify ophthalmologists to practice the procedure. Hospitals and surgery centers that own an excimer laser demand that doctors have a certificate stating they have been trained in a particular procedure. After extensive practice, eye surgeons should perform their first operations on carefully selected individuals and then on the full range of patients under the guidance of a skilled LASIK surgeon.

Nowadays, ophthalmologists from every subspecialty are getting pushed and pulled into refractive surgery. Eye doctors specialize—some study the cornea, some the crystalline lens, and others the retina, for example. But when asked if they intend to do excimer laser surgery, over 97 percent say yes. The neuro-ophthalmologist or the fellow at the university—who hasn't performed surgery in years—says: "Yes, I plan to do refractive surgery." Some physicians perceive that laser procedures are fairly easy to learn. A short procedure, LASIK looks deceptively simple. But, in fact, refractive surgery—especially LASIK—has a steep and endless learning curve. To become expert at any corneal surgery, the ophthalmologist has to do a substantial number of cases.

One might compare mastering LASIK to learning to perform well a complex musical composition by memory. Even a virtuosic pianist must practice endlessly before her brain and fingers working together can make a difficult Chopin *scherzo* sound like the composer intended. Similarly, it takes time for even the most dedicated ophthalmologist to become an accomplished LASIK surgeon. In addition, your doctor must have enough experience to be able to manage any rare complication.

Why is there such a demand among ophthalmologists all over the world to learn PRK and LASIK? It is mainly due to changes in American medicine. Eye doctors, who are making much less money from other surgeries, are getting pushed out of their traditional practices by declining reimbursements and changes in Medicare. With their incomes dropping, they are attracted to refractive surgery—after all, over a quarter of the population is nearsighted, and millions of them are potential refractive surgery patients.

ADVERTISING REFRACTIVE SURGERY

Some clinics advertise their services. Television, radio, and newspaper ads can be educational—but only if they provide accurate information. Unfortunately, some marketing techniques are misleading—often because they tell only part of the story. Refractive surgery is a complicated subject that should be covered in detail to avoid misleading readers. Ads promising that laser surgery patients can "throw away their glasses" or claiming that this procedure is "totally painless" are improper. Patient testimonials also are inappropriate in eye surgery commercials because every patient has a unique healing response. Such deceptive sales efforts are considered unethical by physicians, the Food and Drug Administration (FDA), and the Federal Trade Commission. The best advertisements for refractive surgery present the facts, including the doctors' credentials, without overstating the surgery's potential or guaranteeing perfect results for everyone.

Clinics are never supposed to make unsubstantiated claims about a surgeon's abilities and results. No ophthalmologist should call himself a "world-renowned" refractive surgeon if he has only done a few cases. He should not refer to himself as an "expert" LASIK surgeon if he's done LASIK for only six months. A clinic cannot report LASIK results without an FDA-approved Investigational Device Exemption (IDE) for that study. A doctor who suggests that refractive surgery patients can throw away their glasses will have more dissatisfied patients than the one who explains that these procedures greatly improve vision. Similarly, if a doctor's staff overstates the advantages of an operation, even patients with nearly perfect results may be dissatisfied with their eyesight. Although many people do have 20/20 vision following excimer laser surgery, ethical doctors tell prospective patients: "We are not promising perfect."

Since the excimer is approved specifically for PRK, marketing efforts have focused on this operation, or on "laser" surgery. In the U.S., LASIK is permitted as a "practice of medicine," as long as this "off-label" procedure—which is practiced worldwide—is in the patient's best interests. Some doctors initially performed LASIK under an FDA Investigational Device Exemption and published outcomes. FDA multicenter LASIK trials began as early as 1991, and, over the years, results have improved. Depending on the status of a particular laser, even today a doctor may be unable to say that his machine has been approved by the FDA. As new lasers are developed, each one must be studied.

Some refractive surgery clinics advertise seminars for interested patients. Others work entirely on a referral basis, offering free screenings. Although seminars can be informative, some people sit in the back and never ask questions. A one-on-one consultation with an eye doctor gives patients more opportunity to receive individualized attention. Ethical surgeons address your concerns and never try to rush you into an elective operation. Nor will they promise to "cure your nearsightedness" or offer you a "quick vision fix."

TALKING WITH YOUR DOCTOR'S PATIENTS

Once you have located an experienced refractive surgeon, you might wish to talk with several patients near your age who had a pre-surgical refractive error similar to yours. For example, if you are forty-five years old with -5 diopters of myopia and -1.25 diopters of astigmatism, you can learn a great deal from talking with someone whose correction is in your range, especially if the person is between forty and fifty years old.

Talking with several patients is different from listening to anec-dotal reports. Be careful about putting too much credence in incomplete second- or third-hand information. References either good or bad can be misleading. Obviously, just because young cousin Joe had a "perfect" result with LASIK doesn't mean that fifty-year-old Uncle Frank will also have the same experience. A bad report also can be misleading, although it may be a warning sign. The nature of all surgery is such that even the best doctors occasionally have a poor outcome—just as the same surgeons may have spectacular results. Unfortunately, no operation will ever allow a physician to get perfect results for every single patient.

So if you hear of a poor result, ask questions. Who was the doc-tor? Who was the patient? What happened? Was the problem eventually corrected? But don't waste your time searching for the surgeon who has never had an unhappy patient or a poor result because he hasn't started operating yet.

A SECOND OPINION

Before having any surgery, get a second opinion from another expert. Your ophthalmologist should always be happy for you to get further advice. If you ask for the name of another refractive surgeon, your doctor should be glad to help you find one. Ask her who she would have operate on her eyes. Some patients hesitate to ask a physician for names of other experts. If your eye care specialist becomes upset when you inquire about another surgeon, be wary. You can benefit from a second opinion by a physician knowledgeable about all kinds of refractive surgery.

Once you choose your doctor, it is imperative that the two of you discuss thoroughly your visual needs. Are you a commercial jet pilot whose corrected vision must be 20/20? Are you an editor who reads manuscripts all day? Are you a computer programmer who stares at a computer screen forty or fifty hours a week? The more your doctor knows about you, the better the two of you can pick the best procedure and correction for you.

Refractive surgery is performed at the patient's request. So become as well informed as possible. You should develop a detailed understanding of all of the advantages and drawbacks of the procedures you're considering. Do you thoroughly understand the legally binding, informed-consent form all surgery patients must sign? Your eye doctor should tell you what to expect before, during, and after surgery. She must carefully explain that—as with any surgery—your clinical results are dependent on how you heal, even though with LASIK the inflammatory response is greatly diminished. Ask her about any possible side effects. What are the risks and possible complications? What is the worst possible outcome? What is the second worst?

Keep in mind that vision correction surgery is elective not just for the patient, but also for the doctor. No physician should ever perform a procedure if he doesn't believe the results justify the risks. We once heard a doctor tell a woman that he personally didn't believe in radial keratotomy, but if she really wanted it, he would do it. Well, a few patients will do anything. A surgeon has a clear responsibility not to perform an operation that he doesn't believe in—even if a patient demands it.

YOUR DOCTOR'S EXCIMER LASER AND THE FDA

Your surgeon's understanding of his laser and his experience using it are key to your surgical outcome. In the medical text, *The Art of LASIK,* by Canadian refractive surgeon, Jeffery J. Machat, M.D., and Stephen G. Slade, M.D. (SLACK Inc., 1998), Dr. Machat writes: "Excimer lasers should not be viewed merely as black boxes. Lasers must be understood, not only to achieve superior refractive results but also to avoid complications." In other words, your doctor must have a basic understanding of how the laser works. Ideally, he should be able to make simple repairs. Since lasers are extraordinarily sensitive to the environment, the doctor must know how minor changes in room temperature and humidity affect the laser beam. With LASIK surgery, your physician's working knowledge of the laser's computer software and the mathematically derived surgical tables that determine your refraction is key to your future eyesight.

How important are the brand name and model of your doctor's laser? Since both can have an impact on your surgical result, you should choose a surgeon who uses the latest technology. The newer scanning lasers, which have expanded capabilities over the older broad-beam ones, may offer the best outcomes. If your surgeon has used lasers made by several different manufacturers and various models within each brand, he will gain a working knowledge of each one's unique effect on clinical results. But regardless of how advanced your doctor's laser is, the most significant factor leading to excellent vision is how familiar he is with the model that he is using on your eyes.

American ophthalmology has been at the forefront in developing innovative surgical techniques, leading the way in treating cataracts and retinal disease. The excimer laser was invented, developed, and patented in the U.S. The first cases were performed here. Nevertheless, we initially were a couple of years behind other countries in excimer laser surgery. For the benefit and protection of the American public, lasers have to undergo a meticulous and time-consuming approval process. Under the Medical Devices Act of 1976, the Food and Drug Administration considers lasers experimental devices that require official sanction. The agency also regulates drugs, but not medical procedures. Once medical devices and drugs are approved, they sometimes are used "off label." For example, doctors often advise patients to take aspirin for other purposes than to reduce pain. Originally, the FDA approved the excimer for PRK, but many doctors have used it to perform LASIK—believing that the newer operation is in their patients' best interests.

To pass FDA requirements, upgraded laser models must undergo large, expensive clinical trials sponsored by each laser manufacturer with the cooperation of ophthalmologists. The companies invest tens of millions of dollars in the studies—sponsoring, running, and administering the tests. It took seven years for Summit Technology to get PRK approval for its laser. The original Phase I clinical trials in humans included a small number of blind eyes. These patients were followed for two years. Then the Phase II study on partially and fully sighted eyes began. Eye doctors followed almost two-hundred eyes for two years. Then the Food and Drug Administration permitted Phase III, which studied about seven hundred eyes. Doctors followed these patients for two years before the FDA allowed the data to be presented. Patients had to make many visits to their doctors, both before and after surgery. Each consultation took an hour or more. Post-surgical visits were required the second and third day, then at one week, one month, three months, six months, nine months, one year, eighteen months, and two years. Since extensive studies showed that the excimer was a safe and effective medical device, the findings were presented to an advisory panel.

Composed of ophthalmologists, optometrists, and FDA members, the advisory panel makes recommendations to the FDA. Next, the agency studies the results and the advice of the panel and, with the ophthalmic division of the FDA, makes a final decision. After reviewing the patient data, FDA approval is either granted or denied by a panel of experts.

The excimer lasers approved for PRK have gone through some of the most stringent tests of any medical devices. Requiring no official FDA stamp-of-approval, older technologies such as heart pacemakers, diamond-tipped knives used in RK, and the ophthalmic cutting instruments known as microkeratomes used in LASIK were permitted under a "grandfather" clause. Without doubt, protecting the consumer from unsafe medical devices is a worthy goal. Unfortunately, the downside to regulation is that the costly and lengthy evaluation process delays the entrance of new technology into the U.S. This means that patients outside this country have quicker access to important advances in laser delivery systems than U.S. citizens. Hence, Americans are often treated with less sophisticated lasers than people living in some less economically advantaged countries. To keep abreast of the latest developments in refractive surgery, responsible eye doctors often travel abroad. In order to achieve the best results possible for their patients, physicians must get hands-on experience using state-of-the-art equipment—no matter where it is available.

WHAT DOES THE COST INCLUDE?

In an ideal world, none of us would have to make a decision about the eyesight that we will have for the rest of our lives based on cost. In the real world, however, almost everyone is concerned about medical expenses. Refractive surgery is a consumer-driven, price-sensitive product generally not covered by health insurance. Such elective operations must be paid for in advance. LASIK and PRK are performed on a half-million dollar excimer laser that is costly to maintain. Eventually, the advent of solid-state lasers may help lower some of these costs by reducing maintenance expenses. In 1992, Summit Technology in Waltham, Massachusetts, and VisX Inc. in Santa Clara, California—initially the only two companies selling FDA-approved excimer lasers—created a joint venture and charged surgeons a $250 Pillar Point royalty fee every time they performed a procedure. This licensing fee, which provided much of the laser company's revenue, was passed on to patients, many of whom had saved for several years to afford surgery. At this writing, the individual laser companies charge about $100 per procedure.

Even though eye surgery is expensive, patients almost never talk about the cost after their procedure. Some patients, however, do say: "I'm generally happy with my result, but can you just get this left eye a little better?" In over fifteen years of performing refractive surgery, none of our patients have as yet said, "My operation wasn't worth the cost."

All prospective patients should ask their doctors exactly what the price covers. How much pre-surgical and follow-up care is included in the cost? If you need a refinement or enhancement procedure, is that included? At some clinics, excimer laser surgery is more expensive than RK because LASIK and PRK require more technologically advanced equipment. Other doctors charge the same for RK and laser surgery because they want to eliminate the cost factor from the decision-making process.

Before surgery, one RK patient said, "I price-comparison-shopped before I had RK, and I saved enough money to have my fingernails wrapped in silk for six months." Well, if she received equal value for less money, great. All of us have to be concerned about our finances. We think, however, that since eyesight—which affects every aspect of life—is irreplaceable, informed patients will examine the value they receive for their money. A highly experienced surgical team should increase your odds of an excellent result and decrease the risk of complications. Those patients who no longer need glasses, contact lenses, lens insurance, or cleaning and wetting solutions save on these expenses after surgery.

CHAPTER SEVEN

EXAMINING YOUR EYES

As you focus on each of these words, each
eye swings back and forth a hundred times a
second, and, every second, the retina performs
ten billion computer-like calculations.
                                        —*The Incredible Machine*

A critical element in your decision-making process will be a thorough examination by your doctor who will ask you the detailed questions necessary for a complete medical and ophthalmic history. He will study your ocular health to rule out any pathology that might contribute to your vision problems. Are your corneas and retinas healthy? What is the pressure inside of your eyes? Is it elevated? Do you have ocular hypertension or glaucoma? If you are older, is your crystalline lens starting to cloud, signaling the beginnings of cataracts?

He will want to know your focusing ability and will measure your refractive error. Are you nearsighted or farsighted? Do you have astigmatism, presbyopia, or both? Exactly what is your uncorrected and best-corrected visual acuity (BCVA)? Is your focusing error relatively stable, or do you have to change your glasses prescription significantly every year? How well does your crystalline lens accommodate for near vision? How do your eyes work together? Which one is dominant?

Your doctor will put "cycloplegic" drops in your eyes that temporarily rest the muscles that control the focusing mechanism of your crystalline lens. Such drops also dilate your pupils so that your physician can see inside your eyes. You will recall that if you are farsighted, all or part of your hyperopia may be corrected by your adjustable lens when you are young. Your doctor can measure the magnitude of your full correction when the lens behind your cornea is pharmacologically rendered unable to compensate for hyperopia. Refractive surgeons usually treat all of the hyperopia because, with age, the crystalline lens no longer helps to pull the image forward onto your retina. If you are nearsighted, your physician will need to know the current power of this lens to help you see near objects once your myopia is corrected.

Two patients may both read the 20/30 line on the eye chart, but one might have much better vision than the other. This scale fails to differentiate between the person who quickly reads the letters and numbers and a patient who struggles to see each figure. These two people both have 20/30 visual acuity, but they have much different vision. In other words, quantitatively, their visual acuities measure the same, but qualitatively, they are definitely unequal.

To assess your vision more precisely, scientists have developed the "contrast gradient visual acuity" test. Your eye doctor measures the sensitivity of your visual acuity using various shades of gray. In the real world, objects are seldom black and white—they are shades of colors. Patients never say that they have poor contrast sensitivity. They say: "My vision isn't sharp or crystal clear. I wish it were more crisp."

Your eye doctor will want to assess how well you see in dim light. He will ask if you have a problem with glare at night or in bright light. If you have high myopia, especially if you are young, you may have more potential for glare and halos at night. Your doctor must take many factors into account when studying your case.

Since refractive operations are performed on the cornea, your physician will carefully examine the window of your eye in great detail using highly sophisticated equipment. He will study both eyes through a slit-lamp microscope. When he looks through this instrument, which has a magnification power of six to forty times or more, he can observe the clarity of your corneas. Scars show up, as do changes in the crystalline lens and other parts of the eye. Using special attachments to this instrument, your eye doctor also can focus the microscope on the back, or "fundus," of your eyeball to examine your retina. As your physician views the retinal macula, optic disc, and the nutrient-carrying vascular system, he can pinpoint many abnormalities of the eye.

Your retina reveals not only important information about your ocular health, but about your systemic health as well. A window to the body, the retina is the only place where one can see the pattern of the blood vessels in their natural state. Some vascular diseases are evident on examination of the retina. Scarring of the vessels, hemorrhages, and microaneurysms (tiny "balloon-like" sacs) are apparent. In patients with hypertensive disease or elevated blood pressure, the doctor can see a narrowing of the blood vessels. If a patient has diabetes, the physician often can see the effects of this condition on these vessels.

Your doctor may photograph and evaluate your cornea's vital endothelial layer, which lies near your crystalline lens. Without the metabolic pumping action of this thin layer of cells, your clear cornea would become opaque like the white of your eye. Using a special endothelial microscope attachment, he actually "counts" how many endothelial cells you have per square millimeter. Key to maintaining the partially dehydrated state of the cornea—and thus its clarity—these endothelial cells cannot regenerate. Their density declines significantly with age. Patients with a low endothelial count may not be good candidates for refractive surgery.

Your eye doctor will take the physical measurements of your eye that affect your surgical result. As we explain in detail in chapter 2, key factors influencing the outcome of LASIK are the thickness of your cornea before surgery, the amount of tissue removed by the excimer laser, and the depth of the resculpted cornea. Using ultrasonic pachymetry, your physician can measure corneal depth with astonishing precision. Before surgery, your surgeon will use carefully derived calculations to determine the exact diameter and thickness of the amount of tissue vaporized by the laser. He can monitor your intra-ocular pressure with a special instrument called a "tonometer" to rule out glaucoma.

Mapping Your Cornea

A remarkable innovative technique called "corneal topography" can generate a computer printout that shows the curvature and the "hills and valleys" of your cornea (see fig. 19). By studying these brightly color-coded contour maps, your physician can diagnosis corneal shape abnormalities and monitor changes in the front surface of your eye. A thorough understanding of the various elevations of your eye's bubble-like window can help your doctor decide whether you are a candidate for refractive surgery. If you decide to have LASIK, a specialist can literally take "before and after" pictures that show surgically-induced changes in your corneal topography. Used in evaluating your results, these maps show the pre- and post-surgical dioptric (refractive) power of your cornea. Rare complications usually can be easily pinpointed. For a nearsighted person, such elevation "photos" should show the flattening effect of the operation on the cornea.

To create topography maps of your cornea, high resolution video cameras that are attached to a specially programmed computer photograph your eye's front surface and profile (see fig. 19). Each half-diopter change in elevation, which has a different light-focusing power, is represented by a different shade of color. The steeper curvatures, or "hills," are colored in warm shades of reds, oranges, and yellows while the flatter "valleys" are cool shades of light and dark blue. The middle areas are green. In other words, the steepest elevations with greatest refractive power are bright red and the lowest elevations with the least dioptric power are dark blue.

Kept in your chart, these elevation maps graphically illustrate the different refractive power of many points on your cornea and most irregularities in its surface. Corneal topography helps your doctor see how the pattern of your astigmatism looks on paper. As you now know, this refractive error is often caused by unevenness in the curvature of the cornea's surface. Topographic maps may also enable your physician to rule out subclinical keratoconus (a cone-shaped steepening and thinning of the cornea that causes irregular astigmatism). In addition, he can diagnose subtle conditions with corneal topography that might be missed with less sophisticated tests.

Your eye doctor will compare the astigmatism shown on your corneal maps to the total refractive astigmatism that your glasses correct. You will recall that these measurements don't always agree. As discussed earlier, some astigmatism is caused by irregularities within the eye. Laser surgery corrects only corneal astigmatism. Hence, corneal topography helps your doctor predict how much of your astigmatism can be successfully treated with the laser.

Corneal maps also can help your doctor find the best contact lens fit for you. A computer-generated image of your cornea can quickly "try on" many different types of contact lenses from the computer's large database of soft, soft toric (for astigmatism), and rigid gas permeable lenses without placing a single lens in your eye.

Let's follow Karen as Dr. Baker mapped the topography of the surface of her eyes before her LASIK procedure. He wanted her operation to be based on the most accurate surgical correction data that modern technology could provide. To study the curvature of the window of Karen's eye with corneal topography, Dr. Baker asked her to place her head on the chin rest in front of an instrument called an "image acquisition unit." It looks like a big hollow plastic cone with backlit, target-like rings (doctors call them Placido rings) painted on its concave interior walls (see fig. 19). Some systems also have two scanning slit-lamps attached for more precise and comprehensive measurements. Karen felt absolutely no pain because corneal topography is a totally non-invasive, "no-touch" mapping technique. As she stared at the blinking fixation light in the center of the cone's black and white concentric circles, an image of her eye with the Placido rings reflected on it immediately appeared on the color computer screen. Since the front curvature of Karen's cornea was irregular, the reflected rings appeared distorted. Depending on the system used, the video cameras record images of the eye from one or more angles, and the computer calculates the corneal curvature and elevation data. Other medical information about Karen's eyes was entered in the computer's database.

Within a minute, the computer software generated a color printout showing the curvature and approximate topographic elevations of Karen's cornea. The exact location of the "bow-tie" shaped pattern of her astigmatism was clearly shown (see fig. 19). Unlike many myopic patients, Karen's corneas were not unusually steep; she was nearsighted because the length of each eyeball from front to back is longer than normal.

Even though Karen hadn't worn her disposable contact lenses for a week, the map of the clear front part of her eye still showed a slight amount of lens-induced corneal warpage. Before surgery, Dr. Baker asked Karen not to wear her disposable contacts for a week so that her corneas could resume their natural shape. If she had worn rigid gas permeable lenses, she would have removed them for several weeks or longer before refractive surgery. Right before her operation, Dr. Baker took another reading of the contour of the surface of Karen's eyes to make certain her corneas were no longer distorted from contact lens use. Such pre-operative screenings are essential before any refractive surgery.

After her LASIK operation, Karen's doctor made another topographic map to show how her cornea looked after surgery. Then the computer generated a third map, called a "difference map," that graphically illustrated the profile of the ablated corneal tissue. By studying these colorful printouts, Dr. Baker knew exactly how the operation changed Karen's cornea. He compared her subjective visual acuity as measured by the eye chart with what the post-operative maps of her cornea indicated her vision might be. The two readings don't always agree because of misalignments within the eye leading to astigmatism. For example, if Karen's astigmatism had been caused by irregularities in her crystalline lens, her topographic map would have indicated a different refraction than her subjective eye chart refraction.

CHAPTER EIGHT

WHAT THE LONG, AMAZING HISTORY OF REFRACTIVE SURGERY MEANS TO YOU

"Here lies Salvatore d'Avant, the inventor of spectacles.
May God forgive his sins."
—The Epitaph of Thirteenth century innovator,
Salvatore d'Avant

A BRIEF HISTORY OF RK

In 1973, Svyatoslav N. Fyodorov, M.D., Moscow's Henry Ford of ophthalmology, popularized RK, radial keratotomy, for the correction of nearsightedness. A colorful figure, Dr. Fyodorov is blessed with many diverse talents seldom found in one person: not only is he an innovative surgeon and a creative entrepreneur, Dr. Fyodorov, above all, is an enthusiastic promoter, a master at handling the news media. Svyatoslav, "Slava" to his friends, became intensely interested in RK when the eyesight of a teenage patient improved after he suffered multiple cuts to his cornea. As the story goes, the boy's glasses were broken during a fight. Dr. Fyodorov removed the sharp fragments from the boy's eye. Remarkably, after the wounds healed, the Russian doctor noticed that his young patient could see better.

Twenty years earlier, another surgeon, Professor Tsutomu Sato, had performed RK on Japanese World War II fighter pilots. He hoped to help Japan's war effort against the Allies by improving the soldiers' visual acuity. Unfortunately for thousands of his patients, Sato's primitive RK technique—unlike modern RK—cut too deeply into the cornea. His flawed surgical approach introduced the knife into the cornea not only from the front but also from the back through the anterior chamber. In other words, he made multiple cuts right through the vital endothelial, or the last layer of the cornea. About twenty years after surgery, many of Sato's patients lost vision because the metabolic endothelial pump could no longer maintain the cornea in the partially dehydrated state necessary for clear vision. The doctor died unaware that some of his patients would develop severe complications caused by his operation. Japanese doctors abandoned the technique.

Dr. Fyodorov was familiar with Dr. Sato's earlier work. The Russian doctor knew that if he made cuts on the front surface of the cornea—instead of the back—he could change the corneal curvature without significantly damaging the endothelium. After carefully studying Dr. Sato's work and experimenting on rabbits and other animals, Dr. Fyodorov refined RK, eliminating incisions through the anterior chamber.

Dr. Fyodorov set up clinics all over Russia. Traveling around the Mediterranean on his opulent cruise ship that doubled as an eye hospital, the ophthalmologist has operated on tens of thousands of people on land and at sea.

I first met Dr. Fyodorov when I visited Russia as coordinator of Project Orbis, the DC-10 charity eye hospital (see fig. 25). He took us into his personal office and served everyone caviar. On a table behind his desk were nine old-fashioned black rotary telephones. Each one was on a different line. Since there was no integrated push button communication system, all nine phones could ring at once. Dr. Fyodorov, who has held political office in Russia, would pick up one phone, then the other, and the other, sometimes trying to talk to nine people at the same time.

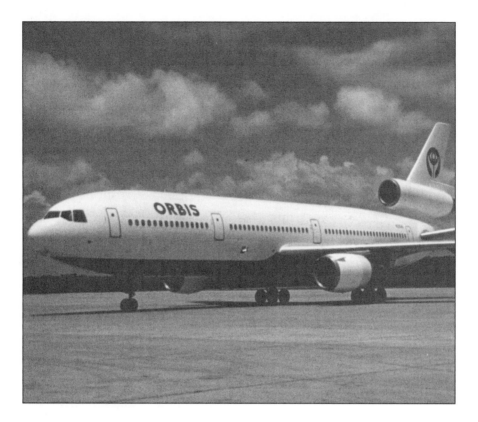

Figure 25
Orbis, the DC-10 charity eye hospital.

A dynamic leader and catalyst for innovation, Dr. Fyodorov surrounded himself with other doctors, engineers, and computer software people. Although he created an environment that fostered the integration of advanced technologies into ophthalmology, his famous assembly line approach to RK made little sense to me. The entire surgical setup was amazing—it looked like a science fiction movie. Since Dr. Fyodorov was paid by the Soviet government on a per-surgery basis, he attempted to speed up the operative process by placing eight people at once on a linear conveyor belt. I watched as the surgical assistants laid the patients down on a series of stretchers on a metal rack and draped each person with white sheets. One of the visitors noted that the patients looked like loaves of bread going into an oven. The operating room door even resembled an oven door. It slid up, the assembly line advanced, a patient went inside, and the door slammed shut.

Looking through a microscope with a video camera attached, each of the five or so attending doctors seated along the human assembly line performed one step of the patient's surgery. Then the table would move so that each patient stopped in front of the next surgeon. Every person's operative eye appeared on a separate TV screen over the surgical suite. Above the operating theater was another room that looked down on the patients. A doctor with a microphone monitored the entire proceedings. After each surgeon completed his part of the operation, he would place the instruments on a tray, which remained with the patient. To indicate that he was finished with that step, the doctor would sit back in his chair. On tracts, the gurneys on the "people-conveyor" advanced when the monitoring physician gave the signal. Patients kept moving between doctors until all of the four to thirty-two RK incisions were completed.

In 1978, Leo D. Bores, M.D., of Detroit, Michigan, brought RK to the United States, using Dr. Fyodorov's surgical technique. Ridiculed by other doctors and the news media, he endured endless grief for popularizing RK in this country. Spencer P. Thornton, M.D., developed the nomograms (the correction codes) and the instrumentation for the operation. J. Charles Casebeer, M.D., whose excellent work standardized RK, taught the technique to many surgeons.

At first, most ophthalmologists, including myself, didn't like the idea of operating on a perfectly healthy eye to correct near-sightedness. I remember the first time I saw an RK patient. As a student at Louisiana State University in New Orleans in the early 1980s, I was doing my residency under Herbert E. Kaufman, M.D., the leading corneal expert in the world. Revolutionizing the treatment of eye disease, he introduced the soft therapeutic contact lens to reduce eye pain. One day while I was working at the Eye Center, I heard the famous ophthalmologist's page: "All residents come to Exam Room Three." He spoke in a gruff voice. We all hurriedly gathered around an RK patient from abroad. The desperate woman had come to New Orleans to see Dr. Kaufman because she was suffering from a disastrous surgical result.

"Look what RK has done to this poor woman's cornea!" said Dr. Kaufman. "This is the most horrible thing you're ever gonna see—this is just terrible!"

After examining the woman's eyes, I remember talking about the case with the other residents. We all agreed that RK was a terrible operation. "How could anyone ever do such a thing to a patient's eye?" I asked. "Can you imagine? Her cornea looks like raw hamburger!" But as Dr. Kaufman started seeing good RK results, he eventually changed his opinion about the operation and began doing it. As more and more patients requested the procedure, the National Eye Institute, a division of the U.S. National Institutes of Health, funded the famous multicenter PERK study to evaluate RK. Chaired by George O. Waring III, M.D., the five-year program, which followed 435 patients, helped define this procedure. Results were published in peer-reviewed ophthalmology journals. Today, RK is no longer considered experimental surgery; it can be a good operation when performed properly for carefully selected patients. (We will discuss the safety, effectiveness, and limitations of RK in detail in chapter 9.)

A BRIEF HISTORY OF PRK

In 1983, Stephen L. Trokel, M.D., an ophthalmologist at Columbia University, revolutionized refractive surgery with a brilliant idea: in a ground-breaking paper published in the *American Journal of Ophthalmology*, he proposed that the excimer laser, which was used to etch circuits in tiny computer microchips, had the potential to treat the human cornea. Dr. Trokel had seen a picture taken by Dr. S.R. Srinivasan of how the excimer could etch smooth notches in a human hair (see fig. 21). Dr. Srinivasan was a physicist at the IBM Thomas J. Watson Research Center in Yorktown Heights, New York. The two doctors collaborated on a work that showed the effect of excimer laser radiation on bovine corneas.

Working with California physicist Charles R. Munnerlyn, Ph.D., Dr. Trokel started the extensive research that eventually led to modern laser surgery for vision correction. An optical engineer, Dr. Munnerlyn formulated the computer vision correction codes upon which PRK is based. These mathematically derived algorithms—which are a key to successful results—show how much tissue should be removed to correct a particular degree of nearsightedness. Marguerite B. McDonald, M.D., a renowned corneal surgeon, conducted animal studies at Louisiana State University that indicated that Dr. Trokel's original theory was correct. Electron micrographs graphically showed that, unlike the other lasers used in ophthalmology, the cool excimer laser left the surrounding corneal tissue virtually undisturbed. The excimer could remove corneal cells, predictably changing the dome-like curvature of the window of the eye.

In 1987, the doctors began PRK studies on blind human eyes. The results were encouraging. The same year in Berlin, Theodore W. Seiler, M.D., Ph.D., performed the first excimer laser treatment on a normally sighted eye. In 1988, Dr. McDonald and Dr. Kaufman performed the first PRK procedure with the excimer laser in the U.S. Rigorous, carefully documented clinical trials on sighted eyes commenced throughout the United States. Finally, in October 1995, the FDA approved Summit Technology's excimer laser for PRK to correct nearsightedness. In March 1996, a laser developed by VISX Corporation received FDA approval. By this time, the excimer had been used extensively throughout the world to treat nearsightedness.

I first heard about refractive laser eye surgery when I was studying under Dr. Kaufman at Louisiana State University. "Well," said the eminent surgeon, "don't worry about having to learn RK because it will be replaced by laser surgery. The patients will just come in, and the laser will treat their nearsightedness maybe even while they are reading a magazine. Afterwards, they will get up, walk out, and see perfectly."

Such was the dream! Unfortunately, fulfilling this prophesy hasn't been easy. Eye doctors had hoped that the original laser-based PRK procedure would be the answer to the prayer for the "perfect refractive surgery." But even though this procedure has helped many people, as we emphasize throughout this book, PRK has failed to live up to all our expectations.

Of the refractive operations, LASIK comes closest to achieving this goal. The surgeon carefully enters the patient's targeted correction into the computer. The machine's software calculates the number of pulses required, and the laser removes a pre-determined amount of tissue. But, although LASIK is highly automated in many respects, even this advanced surgical technique is far from a "push-button" operation, at least from the doctor's point of view. Management of the protective flap created from corneal tissue, as emphasized throughout this book, requires great finesse.

A BRIEF HISTORY OF LASIK

The story of the evolution of the modern LASIK procedure began about fifty years ago. In 1949, Jose I. Barraquer, M.D., of Bogota, Colombia, the father of lamellar refractive surgery, suggested that refractive defects could be diminished by operating within the layers of the cornea. Even though doctors had been splitting the cornea to remove scars for hundreds of years, the idea of operating on a healthy eye to correct refractive errors was considered radical. Experimenting with animals for thirteen years, Dr. Barraquer developed many of the theories behind modern vision correction surgery. He called his new surgical technique "refractive keratoplasty," meaning plastic surgery for optical purposes.

A scientific giant, Dr. Barraquer invented much of the original ophthalmic equipment that has been updated for today's vision correction procedures. One of his many contributions to refractive surgery was the first hand-driven microkeratome to cut the cornea. Based on the design of a carpenter's plane, this blade-bearing instrument advanced his surgical technique beyond freehand dissections of the cornea. In 1963, he first used the microkeratome to treat nearsighted and farsighted patients.

In the book *Lamellar Refractive* Surgery by J. Charles Casebeer, M.D., Luis A. Ruiz, M.D., and Stephen G. Slade, M.D., Dr. Casebeer explains:

> At first I used my formulas and an electronic calculator to determine the exact surgical action for each case, but later this was replaced by my computer software calculations. In the early years, I made *corneal lenticulas* [refractive disks honed from actual corneal tissue] with a manually driven contact lens lathe with CO_2 circuits attached to freeze the tissue.

In other words, to correct severe nearsightedness, Dr. Barraquer surgically removed a slice of the patient's cornea, froze and milled the tissue on a contact lens cryolathe, and returned the thawed living tissue to the front of the person's eye. Stitches held the resculpted lens in place. Even though many of Dr. Barraquer's patients showed improvement in unaided visual acuity, doctors abandoned the technique of freezing corneal disks because it damaged the tissue. Although such procedures seem almost archaic by today's standards, many of Dr. Barraquer's ideas were years ahead of his time. He taught doctors how to operate within the inner layers of the cornea while preserving the top layers (the epithelium and Bowman's membrane).

The contributions of many other refractive surgeons have made LASIK possible. A colleague of Dr. Barraquer's, Luis A. Ruiz, M.D.—who has performed tens of thousands of refractive procedures—was the first to do a "double-cut" operation that doctors call "keratomileusis in situ." During this surgery, Dr. Ruiz removed a round, corneal cap, placing the thin tissue in a special container. To flatten the cornea, he then cut and discarded a second, smaller, plano disc (one with no curvature or power) from the patient's exposed corneal bed. Next, he carefully replaced the cap, securing it with tiny stitches. Dr. Ruiz performed this operation *by hand*, manually moving the blade-containing microkeratome across the cornea. Keep in mind that this surgical instrument looks like a tiny carpenter's plane. Although many patients showed improvement in visual acuity without corrective lenses, results lacked the accuracy of today's excimer laser surgery.

In the late 1980s, Dr. Ruiz vastly improved lamellar corneal surgery by *automating* the microkeratome, leading to an operation called "automated lamellar keratoplasty," or ALK. Up to this time, these procedures lacked the predictability of modern LASIK mainly because the hand-driven microkeratome could be an imprecise instrument. Few doctors had the skill to move the keratome manually across the cornea at the constant speed and pressure necessary to produce an excellent outcome.

ALK allowed refractive surgeons to help severely nearsighted people who were too myopic to have RK. ALK, which introduced many ophthalmologists to lamellar corneal surgery, offered better and more stable results than RK for these patients. Correcting severe myopia with RK required too many incisions. With ALK, both cuts were mechanically controlled, and the operation was relatively safe. Patients' eyes looked nice the day after surgery, and people quickly got final results. Although the automated keratome greatly improved results, the procedure still lacked the accuracy that patients and their doctors desired. ALK was extremely dependent on surgical technique. An ALK study in 1993 reported that 70 percent of patients had uncorrected visual acuity of 20/40 or better after surgery, while 97 percent could at least read the 20/200 line on the eye chart. With the discovery of modern LASIK and other techniques, eye doctors have abandoned ALK, although it may still be used for patients with greater than -14 diopters of myopia who cannot have LASIK.

The merger of two technologies, automated keratomileusis in situ and the computer-controlled excimer laser, finally brought us LASIK. Working under a surgical flap, surgeons treated the inner cornea with the computer software-guided excimer laser. This technique achieved much more accurate results than ALK. In 1989, Lucio Buratto, M.D., of Milan, Italy, used the excimer to remove tissue from the *underside* of a free corneal cap. In 1990, Dr. Theo Seiler published his earlier results of treating the surgically exposed inner cornea with the excimer laser in both blind and sighted patients. In 1991, Iaonnis Pallikaris, M.D., of Keraklion, Crete, began studies on sighted human eyes, using a combination of a specially engineered, manually advanced microkeratome and the excimer laser. Dr. Pallikaris coined the term "LASIK," which as you recall stands for "laser in situ keratomileusis," also sometimes called "laser intra-stromal keratomileusis."

In 1991, working with Dr. Stephen F. Brint under a Summit Technology investigational protocol, we performed the first modern LASIK procedure as it is currently practiced. After creating a protective hinged corneal flap with the mechanically advanced, geared microkeratome, I used the excimer laser to remove tissue from the newly exposed inner corneal bed. I carefully put the flap back in place. It served as a natural bandage over the treated area. LASIK is still performed this way all over the world. The precision of the microkeratome's corneal shaper allows surgeons to cut protective flaps of precisely pre-determined thickness and diameter, leading to the increased accuracy of the procedure. Along with Dr. Luis Ruiz, Dr. Charles Casebeer, and others, we developed and improved the mathematical calculations, or nomograms, upon which LASIK is based. We worked to standardize the procedure to try to avoid intra-operative complications. Producing excellent results in the U.S. under FDA research protocols, LASIK currently is our most advanced vision correction surgery.

A few years ago, while I was having breakfast at the American Academy of Ophthalmology with my friend, Dr. George O. Waring III, we speculated about what people might call the new LASIK procedure. I came up with the idea of nicknaming it "flap and zap" surgery. We immediately decided, however, that even though these terms are rather descriptive, they inadvertently trivialize a life-changing operation. Although we no longer refer to LASIK in this way, we did mention this nickname to a couple of other doctors, and eventually some people did start calling the procedure "flap and zap" surgery.

As this brief history shows, the state-of-the-art in refractive eye surgery is continually evolving. Supported by the scientific community, doctors are always looking for better ways to solve their patients' problems. When a new procedure is first developed, surgeons are faced with a difficult dilemma. We wonder, "Should we stop doing an older operation that we know well and start learning this latest technique?" "Will it really provide the best possible outcome for our patients?" Refractive surgery candidates go through a rather similar thought process. They ask themselves: "Should I have this operation now, or should I wait a few years in hopes that results will improve?" Most people who have LASIK now can still have further treatment later, although the risks are higher with repeat surgery.

CHAPTER NINE

OLDER NON-LASER OPERATIONS: RK AND AK

*Constantly considering new ideas, an accomplished eye
surgeon must be committed to use new and old techniques
in order to offer the best chance of success for his patients.*
—R. Bruce Grene, M.D.

For years, more people had RK (radial keratotomy) to correct nearsightedness than any other vision correction operation. Continuously mired in heated controversy, radial keratotomy was the first refractive surgical procedure. Considering its varied reputation, you may wonder if RK has served patients well. The answer depends on whom you ask. People with excellent results call it the best thing that ever happened to them. They enthusiastically recommend RK to their friends. Patients who were over- or undercorrected or who had other complications may wish that they had waited for better technology.

Debating the merits of operating on a healthy cornea to improve vision, some eye doctors took either a "pro" or "anti" position toward radial keratotomy. Others assumed a wait-and-see approach. Many specialists objected to bending the cornea to refocus the eye. Nevertheless, as results improved, even conservative physicians recognized the value of RK. After the 1984 National Eye Institute PERK study, the American Academy of Ophthalmology lifted the experimental status of RK, finding it safe and effective for mild to moderate myopia.

Largely replaced now by laser surgery, RK usually provided good results with the lower ranges of nearsightedness. In fact, many RK patients achieved visual outcomes almost on par with those available today with the newer operations. Patients with severe myopia and astigmatism had the least satisfactory results. In fact, most RK problems occurred because doctors pushed the procedure past its technological limits—treating the higher ranges of myopia or refining primary results with multiple operations. Most doctors now do not consider radial keratotomy the best treatment for large amounts of refractive error.

Since LASIK is a better option for almost all patients, who might be a candidate for RK? People with mild myopia who are unable to have a LASIK keratectomy still have the option of considering modern radial keratotomy or PRK. Some patients have an orbital anatomy that precludes LASIK. For example, if the eyes are unusually small, the surgeon may be unable to fit on the suction ring. That patient can still be treated with four-cut mini-RK, a modified surgical technique with short incisions. I only correct under -3 diopters of myopia with mini-RK. Doctors perform a related operation called "astigmatic keratotomy" (AK) that uses "T-cuts" or "arcs" to flatten the cornea's steepest, most powerful refractive meridian, (see fig. 8). In some cases, AK can be a good enhancement tool for mild residual astigmatism after LASIK. RK has not been successfully adapted to treat farsightedness.

Though most RK patients would "do it again," some have visual symptoms or optical aberrations after surgery. Acutely aware that they needed better ways to correct poor vision, eye doctors searched for ways to improve surgical techniques. With the advent of LASIK, ophthalmologists now have a safer and more accurate way to treat nearsightedness.

PHYSIOLOGICAL EFFECTS OF RK ON THE EYE

If you are considering radial keratotomy, you should understand its physiological effects on the eye. Causing the cornea to bend, this procedure's mechanism of action is totally different from LASIK or PRK. Unlike laser surgery, radial keratotomy works by weakening the mid-periphery of the cornea. Looking through the operating microscope, an RK surgeon attempts to improve vision by cutting tiny radial or spoke-like incisions in the cornea with a guarded diamond-tipped knife (see fig. 8). The normal pressure inside the eye pushes against the surgically weakened portion of the cornea, causing it to bow out over the incised area in a knee-like bend (at about 7 millimeters). As the unsutured incisions expand outward, the central cornea flattens, almost as if tissue were removed. When the incisions heal, light should fall nearer the retina.

RK patients treated for mild nearsightedness look at the world through a central uncut "clear zone," and the incisions do not extend through the visual axis, or line-of-sight. Generally, people are unaware of these incision scars. Unfortunately, however, patients treated for high myopia may see the RK scars, especially when the pupil dilates at night. In fact, even some mildly nearsighted patients notice the healed incisions if they have big pupils that dilate beyond the incision-free clear zone. The more relaxing incisions the surgeon makes, and the deeper and longer they are—the more the cornea flattens. Of these surgical variables, the size of the clear zone is the most crucial consideration determining the amount of myopia treated.

Radial keratotomy refocuses the eye, but it is still technically considered myopic because the length of the eyeball remains unchanged. You will recall that most nearsighted eyes are elongated. Hence, even if you achieve perfect 20/20 visual acuity after RK, you still have the same chance of retinal detachment or separation of the layers of the retina as you did before the operation.

RESULTS

Following radial keratotomy, 93 percent of patients achieve 20/40 visual acuity and 54 percent attain 20/20. In *Refractive Keratotomy*, George O. Waring III writes: "The best we can do [with RK] is to predict that the result is likely to fall within a particular range of outcomes. Most published reports have indicated a precision for predicting the refractive outcome [of RK] of about plus or minus 2D [2 diopters] for 80 to 90 percent of eyes."

Such results depend not only on the degree of myopic error and the surgical technique, but also on the way each individual heals. Age affects wound-healing response. A seventy-year-old—who has a less aggressive wound-healing response and heals slower than a younger person—attains about twice as much effect as a thirty-year-old. Although doctors know that biological age affects how the incisions heal, chronological age may vary from biological age—leading to an occasional unexpected outcome.

The condition of your collagen is one important factor determining how your cornea heals. You can do an informal test that might indicate how "young" your collagen connective tissue is: if you twist a fold of skin above your knuckle, and then let go, you can observe how quickly the pinched skin falls back into place. In theory, the better your collagen, generally the faster the fold fades away. Of course, your weight, fitness level, and other factors may also influence your result. Since people of the same numerical age grow old at varying rates, their collagen and their healing response will differ. After RK, the cornea—which is made of collagen—will heal more slowly, depending in part on your biological age.

According to ophthalmologist Spencer P. Thornton, M.D., "By careful pre-operative planning and by following the nomogram (correction code) precisely, doctors can come very close to the targeted result in all but a few cases in which unforeseen biological variables [healing rates] produce variation."

ADVANCES IN RK

Although a scalpel will never have the precision of an excimer laser, modern radial keratotomy has evolved into a fairly advanced procedure. If you decide to have it, you will benefit from the efforts of many dedicated scientists who, over the years, have struggled to improve results. When doctors first performed radial keratotomy, they operated with metal blades. Today, surgeons use exquisitely sharp, diamond-tipped blades that make extremely fine incisions. The length of the blade, critical to good post-surgical vision, is now set with a built-in micrometer calibrated to one *millionth* of a meter. With the invention of ultrasonic pachymetry, surgeons can measure the thickness of your cornea more accurately. Nowadays, readings are taken by passing a painless pulse from an ultrasonic transducer to Descemet's membrane (the fourth layer of the cornea) and back to the instrument. Excellent visual results depend on extremely precise calculations of the cornea's depth. Blade length is set based on the thickness of the window of the eye.

If you have radial keratotomy, your doctor will base your operation on calculations derived from sophisticated computerized tables. These mathematical computations will help your surgeon choose the best optical zone size for your particular eyes, considering your age and correction. Developed after years of studying past results with other patients, these surgical tables are more accurate than the ones used to calculate the power of intra-ocular lenses after cataract surgery.

Eye doctors now have observed RK's impact on nearsighted people for many years. They have witnessed how patients perceive their surgical outcomes—how this procedure has thrilled and disappointed people. Scientific studies of results over the past twenty years should help your doctor counsel you. It is easy to forget the importance of such empirical evidence in medicine: reality dictates that, if you are the first person to have a new procedure, you won't benefit from the knowledge gained by earlier patients. On the other hand, if you have an operation performed on thousands, you will benefit from the facts gained from all those who came before you. Accordingly, your doctor would attempt to predict your outcome based on results with cases similar to yours.

Even though the RK consultation process has become more elegant, it still is far from perfect. Each individual's particular outcome is based on a highly educated guess, although experience has improved the *overall* predictability of the procedure. Since every person's healing response is unique, occasionally someone will have a completely unforeseen reaction to RK. In fact, a major reason we recommend LASIK instead of RK or PRK is that the inflammatory wound-healing response is diminished—making the visual outcome more predictable.

THE IMPORTANCE OF SURGICAL TECHNIQUE

If you have RK, your doctor's surgical technique will be absolutely crucial to your visual results. There is little room for error with eye surgery. The keys to your future vision are the *diameter* of the clear zone and the depth and number of incisions (see fig. 8). Keep in mind that the untouched clear zone is the center of the cornea, where no incisions are made. To re-emphasize, the size of this area is the most significant surgical factor determining the amount of your refractive change following RK. The smaller the clear zone (the longer the incisions)—the greater the amount of surgically-induced correction. Although doctors sometimes call the clear zone the optical zone, in reality, they are different. After RK, you would look through a larger area, or optical zone, than the uncut clear zone. Unfortunately, patients with small optical zones are more likely to have glare and halos around lights—which interfere with night driving. A recent surgical technique uses incisions that don't extend as far into the periphery of the cornea. Such modifications can reduce complications associated with RK, such as intra-operative bleeding and corneal instability.

The second most important surgical consideration influencing the degree of refractive change is the *depth* of the incisions. Always remember that a predetermined amount of cornea must be incised to achieve an accurate surgical result. The deeper the slits, the more the cornea flattens. To maintain corneal stability, however, your surgeon must leave a vital amount of uncut supporting corneal tissue. Usually, once blade depth is set, it is not changed. Human corneas are about 720 microns near the edge and about 540 microns in the center. (Remember that one micron equals one millionth of a meter.) Since the eye's window is deeper close to its edges, more uncut corneal bed remains near the white of the eye than near the pupil. To achieve the desired effect, the incisions generally penetrate through 85 to 90 percent of the cornea, almost to Descemet's membrane, the fourth layer. Incisions that cut through less than 75 percent of the cornea are ineffective and can result in severe undercorrection or, eventually, in total regression.

The third key factor influencing your surgical correction is the number of incisions: generally, the more incisions, the greater refractive correction—although, as their number increases, their individual effect decreases. In the 1980s, eight-cut surgery became standard. Today, with laser technology, four-cut radial incisions are generally standard, using a minimum clear zone of four millimeters. RK works best for -1 to -3 diopters of mild nearsightedness.

THE IMPORTANCE OF GOOD CLINICAL JUDGMENT

To meet your expectations, your ophthalmologist must be both an excellent surgeon and a good clinician. If you have RK, your result will not only depend on your doctor's ambidextrous eye-hand coordination, but also on his operative judgment. A doctor can have fantastic hands and produce perfect RK incisions, but if he lacks keen clinical judgment, your visual outcome can be unsatisfactory. Beyond good form, what counts is excellent function—how well you can read the eye chart. Your surgeon must try to customize RK to your individual case, not fit your eyes to the operation.

Keeping a close watch on clinical results leads to a conservative approach to RK. The doctor cannot always go for the "home run" if his patients are to have consistently good outcomes. Part of the intrinsic problem with RK is that, to achieve the desired effect, the surgeon must incise and bend the cornea. An aggressive approach that attempts to correct higher amounts of nearsightedness requires more incisions farther into the clear zone than RK for low myopia. Too much surgery for a particular patient's eye may lead to overcorrection, corneal instability, and fluctuating vision—no matter how straight the incisions are. As you now know, a critical amount of supportive tissue must remain uncut to obtain excellent, fairly stable results. Unfortunately, even when treated conservatively with short incisions, people who appear to be good RK candidates— even those with mild myopia who often have spectacular outcomes—can occasionally become farsighted. RK patients with this problem now can be treated with customized hyperopic LASIK.

An eminent refractive surgeon, Lee Nordon, M.D., explains, "RK appears quite easy, but it is extremely difficult. Surgeons who perform RK incorrectly inappropriately conclude that the procedure does not work; however, those who do it correctly receive more appreciation from their patients than they have ever received in the past."

WHO MIGHT BE A CANDIDATE FOR RK?

As with any refractive operation, before you can determine whether you're a good candidate for RK, you need a clear reading of your own expectations and careful explanations of all the benefits and the short- and long-term risks of this procedure. After RK, you probably hope to see as well without contact lenses as you did with them, and that's a reasonable expectation. If you cannot have LASIK—and if you have low myopia—you may still be able to have RK. Good results will depend on your age, intra-ocular pressure, and sex—and on your doctor's surgical judgment and operative technique. You must be counseled that your outcome won't be totally predictable and that an enhancement procedure might be necessary. In other words, you may need another operation to attempt to achieve an outcome that satisfies you. You must remember, however, that with enhancement surgery, the rewards are less and the risks are much greater than with the first procedure. If you have a less-than-excellent result, you will still need glasses or contact lenses. Fitting contact lenses may be more difficult after RK surgery. In addition, if both of your eyes are focused for the distance, you probably will need reading glasses when you get older. Surgically induced monovision, that is, leaving one eye undercorrected for near vision, can be demonstrated with contact lenses.

United States Army regulations say that the visual demands of active duty, and, more dramatically, the military aviator, are incompatible with RK. In fact, the U.S. military has a blanket policy for all branches of service to disqualify all potential recruits who have had RK. The recruits can still enter their chosen branch with a waiver that exempts the military from responsibility to any future damage to the operative eye. Anyone in a profession with a high risk for trauma to the eyes should probably avoid RK. Fighter pilots, who undergo rapid changes in G-force, can experience fluctuations in vision. The military doesn't want the taxpayers' multi-million dollar airplanes piloted by someone with unpredictable visual acuity.

Most doctors are extremely hesitant to perform radial keratotomy on patients with diabetes. Other medical conditions that can keep people from having RK are an active infection, pregnancy, keratoconus, irregular astigmatism, a history of herpes simplex, corneal inflammatory disease, and correctable visual acuity worse than 20/40. The refractive error should be stable, ideally changing less than 0.5 diopter over an eighteen-month period. RK can undercorrect marijuana users because the illegal drug can lower intra-ocular pressure.

Many patients have health insurance that has failed to keep up with the latest technological advances in eye medicine. Such policies may pay for radial keratotomy but not laser surgery. Some doctors will still do eight-incisional RK for people with such coverage. Patients should understand, however, that LASIK is superior to RK because of the long-term effects on the eye and the accuracy of the procedure. Nevertheless, if the refractive error falls within the RK treatment range, good results are possible. Another option would be to postpone refractive surgery until one can afford LASIK—which probably is the better choice.

THE RK SURGICAL PROCEDURE

If you decide to have RK, here is generally what will happen: RK is a quick procedure performed in a sterile environment with the aid of an operating microscope and ultrasound measuring devices. Before surgery, your doctor will give you a sedative to relax you and put anesthetic and anti-inflammatory drops in your eyes. You'll be covered with a surgical drape. Without your glasses, the operating room may seem dark. Lying on your back under the microscope, you will hear your surgeon talking about the different measurements that will affect your future vision. He is triple-checking every calculation. After your physician positions the operating microscope and applies the lid-specula, he will ask you to stare at the light so that he can mark the center of your new optical zone. You must fixate on the light throughout the rest of the surgery.

Looking through the microscope, your doctor can see the "saccadic," or tiny involuntary movements, of your living eye. Now you will see the instruments come close to your face. Your vision may blur. Your doctor will put more topical anesthetic drops in your eye. He takes some time to remeasure the thickness of your cornea with an ultrasonic pachymeter. You hear some beeping noises, and you sense the instrument touch your eye.

If you have astigmatism, your doctor will gently mark the location and length of the transverse astigmatic incisions. Next, he will identify the central clear zone—the center section of your cornea that remains untouched by the scalpel. Generally speaking, the size of the clear zone is related to the amount of correction attempted. Now your doctor takes a minute or two to mark the precise positions of the four radial cuts. You'll hear him talking about some more numbers as he sets the knife length with a blade micrometer. Examining the knife under the high magnification of a special Micron Scope, your surgeon carefully verifies that the blade length is correct. The blade is accurate to plus or minus five microns, or five one-millionths of a meter in either direction. Excess fluid is removed from the surgical field. Now you'll sense something up very close to your eye. The knife is so near your eye that you cannot see it. It's rather like holding your hand right in front of your eyes; you see the movement and the different shadows. Then the incisions are made. You don't feel them. They don't take much time. In fact, it takes less time to make the incisions than to mark their position on the eye.

The surgery is over. Your doctor will inspect your eye, place broad spectrum antibiotic drops in it, and remove the lid specula and the drape. You'll sit up. Your eyes may feel gritty. Although you may be slightly dazzled for the first minutes by the microscope light, you should see pretty well after surgery. You probably will be able to see the dark numbers of the clock on the operating room wall.

Although some people have severe pain following RK, let's say that you only experience slight discomfort. To keep the pain from getting worse, you immediately take the prescribed pain medications. Pain is controlled best when it is mild. You also use special anti-inflammatory eye drops to reduce the release of "prostaglandins," the fatty acids that can make the eye hurt. At home, you take a sleeping pill and head for your bed. Your friend brings you a small sandwich so you won't wake up hungry and uncomfortable in the middle of the night.

Next morning you feel well enough to reread your post-operative instructions: no make-up near your eyes for at least two weeks; no swimming or sitting in hot-tubs until the doctor says you can.

According to one forty-five-year-old RK patient, "The surgery hurt a lot for about a day or two, but I'd do it over again in a second. I had four diopters of nearsightedness in both eyes before my operation. I have allergies, and I found contact lenses uncomfortable. Since my RK operation, I've had ten years of incredible 20/15 vision, although my eyesight isn't perfect at night. Car headlights seem to have bright starbursts around them, but I consider this a small price to pay for the joy of great daytime vision.

"For the last three years, I have had to wear glasses to read. They really irritate me. If I were still nearsighted, I probably could see up close by just taking off my glasses. My doctor tells me that I might be better off, now that I'm older, if I were *slightly* undercorrected in one eye. My friend had an inexperienced surgeon do her RK. She is extremely unhappy. Her final vision after RK is 20/80 *with glasses*."

THE BODY'S WOUND-HEALING RESPONSE

The eye tries to keep its surface smooth. So about three hours after RK surgery, the epithelial cells near the incisions migrate toward the slits. Within a day or two the cells start to divide, covering the cut. Forming a thin plug in the wound, the epithelial cells travel to the bottom of each incision, totally filling the slit in about one week. Normally, over time new collagen formation in the wound pushes the epithelial plug from the incision, eventually forming a thin scar. Most RK wounds are healed after three to six months. In some cases, a large epithelial plug forms.

As mentioned earlier, people heal differently. For older patients, the wound-healing response is reduced, and they heal more slowly than younger patients. Older people thus experience a greater effect from the same amount of surgery than younger people. As a result, patients over forty have a higher risk of becoming hyperopic after RK.

WHAT COULD GO WRONG?

Radial keratotomy can have side effects that usually resolve over time and complications that permanently affect the surgical results. Many nearsighted RK patients experience a planned initial overcorrection causing farsightedness, but after the healing period their vision usually improves. Unfortunately, some people remain overcorrected. Others have residual uncorrected nearsightedness. RK patients also can still become more nearsighted with time if their eyeball naturally elongates. Myopic regression from corneal steepening, however, is less of a problem following radial keratotomy than after PRK. As discussed in detail in the chapter on enhancements, RK patients with a significant residual error often can have further treatment with LASIK—if their incisions are well-healed and their corneas are stable.

People sometimes complain about the quality of their eyesight after RK. Remember, we have a good way to measure visual acuity, but we lack precise methods of assessing quality of vision. Individuals can be focused so that they can read the 20/20 line of the eye chart and still have visual problems. Patients may have glare, light sensitivity (photophobia), or starbursts such as streaks of light radiating from street lamps that affect night vision. The size of the incision-free clear zone can impact the quality of vision. Most people who have starbursts, glare, and halos have a 3-millimeter or smaller clear zone. When their eyes dilate, they look through the central portions of these incisions. Diamond-tipped blades, which create finer scars, and anti-inflammatory eye drops have helped reduce glare.

Such side effects are particularly a problem for people with high myopia or astigmatism and for those with dry eyes or large pupils. Persons over forty may have more prominent scarring around the incisions that scatters the light. As the scars heal and become finer, starbursts can diminish, but they may not completely disappear. A small clear zone or too many radial incisions for a particular eye might increase the likelihood of these side effects.

Nowadays, doctors attempt to limit such side effects by performing mini-RK, using only four, half-length incisions. Unfortunately, even the new surgical techniques have not totally eliminated the problems associated with the older RK operations. Some patients still complain of light sensitivity, glare, and starbursts.

To avoid important intra-operative complications, as well as to achieve an excellent result, your doctor must take *extremely* precise measurements of the thickness of your cornea. If the blade nicks the last corneal layer, piercing the eye's anterior chamber, the patient will have a complication known as a "microperforation" of the cornea. The surgeon must vigilantly watch for droplets of aqueous fluid that percolate to the surface when the anterior chamber is accidentally entered. A tiny slit should reseal itself spontaneously, but a larger cut through the cornea, called a "macroperforation," is a serious complication. It may require a stitch to keep the integrity of the anterior chamber intact. The eye must be soaked in antibiotics and patched shut. The RK surgery is aborted.

Every precaution is taken to avoid infections following RK because they can threaten the patient's sight. If an RK patient has atypical redness or pain, the doctor must be called immediately. All infections are dangerous. They must be closely monitored and are treated with antibiotics and steroids.

Some RK patients have fluctuating vision that can change 1 to 2 diopters during the day. People complain of changes in their vision because the cornea is unstable—it keeps moving. The changing pressure inside the eye can cause visual acuity to vary from 20/20 in the morning to 20/60 or worse in the evening. Since the pressure is higher in the morning, the cornea bows out more at the sides, increasing the surgical effect so that the center of the cornea is flatter. This means that someone with residual myopia generally will see better early in the day, while someone with an overcorrection will have clearer vision as the day progresses. The more aggressive the RK surgery, the greater the risk of fluctuating vision.

So will your vision stay put? That's a key question, because radial keratotomy gets results by weakening the mid-peripheral portion of the cornea and permanently changing its shape by causing it to bend. In a way, RK is like throwing a forward pass in a football game. Three things can happen, and two of them are bad: the cornea can bend too much, which can result in overcorrection, or it may bend too little, which will create an undercorrection. Or the cornea can bend just the right amount and stay put, causing a great result. A good RK surgeon can change the shape of the cornea according to a specified plan, but the final results depend on more than operative technique. Thrown into the equation is the patient's wound-healing characteristics—and everybody is different.

Another risk that RK surgeons worry about is irregular astigmatism. By carefully screening refractive surgery candidates, eye doctors can decrease the incidence of this problem. If your cornea is scarred or unstable, you should not have radial keratotomy. To avoid the fine wrinkling of irregular astigmatism, the surgeon must place the tiny incisions skillfully and with great care so that the corneal surface remains smooth after surgery.

Consecutive Hyperopia

Over time, some RK patients become farsighted if the cornea continues to flatten. Called "consecutive hyperopia" by eye doctors, unplanned hyperopic shift can occur if the cornea is unstable after radial keratotomy. In other words, this year a patient's correction may be +1 diopter, next year +2 diopters and nine months later +3 diopters. To try to prevent this problem, most refractive surgeons set limits on the amount of surgery they will perform on someone's eye. As mentioned earlier, doctors have learned to avoid treating the higher ranges of myopia with RK. Correcting severe nearsightedness with RK can require overly long incisions for a particular eye. The goal is to limit corneal instability that sometimes leads to fluctuating vision and eventually even to farsightedness. In fact, the main reason ophthalmologists now usually perform four-incisional mini-RK is to try to prevent the post-operative development of hyperopic shift. Although such new RK surgical techniques have reduced this problem, they have not totally eliminated it.

In his 1,325-page book, *Refractive Keratotomy*, George O. Waring III, M.D., writes, "No clear 'histopathologic' explanation [a study of the cellular pathology] has been offered for the continued increase in effect of surgery in approximately 20 percent of eyes after radial keratotomy. Presumably, the wounds stretch enough to produce more corneal flattening."

ENDOTHELIAL CELL LOSS

As we age, the number of our irreplaceable endothelial cells naturally declines. Probably any trauma to the eye—including radial keratotomy, cataract surgery, or long-term contact-lens wear—has the potential to cause increased loss of endothelial cells, which make up the cornea's last layer, the endothelium. Pumping excess fluid from the eye's window, the endothelium keeps the cornea transparent. The more RK surgery performed on the eye, the higher the incidence of loss of these cells. Eyes with larger RK clear zones usually show much less damage to these cells than corneas with smaller clear zones. If the surgical blade perforates the endothelium into the eye's front fluid-filled chamber, endothelial cells can be lost. The probability of damage to the endothelium increases with repeat RK surgery.

Cataract Surgery after RK

Some people who had radial keratotomy about twenty years ago are now returning to their ophthalmologist to have cataract surgery. These patients, now in their sixties, are starting to reach the age where their crystalline lens naturally begins to cloud. Most cataracts can be successfully removed after incisional surgery. The actual surgical technique to remove cataracts is the same for RK patients and for untreated eyes. The cataract surgeon will ask for the original pre-RK measurements of the eye. The calculations to set the refractive power of the intra-ocular lens are more complex after radial keratotomy because the cornea has been reshaped. Nevertheless, in expert hands, post-RK cataract surgery results are about the same as those for people who have never had vision correction surgery.

Fitting Contact Lenses after RK

If you are considering radial keratotomy, remember that fitting contacts may become more difficult afterwards. RK changes the cornea's profile. You may have to wear rigid lenses rather than soft contacts if you have residual myopia, if you regress, or if you develop hyperopia or astigmatism. The risk of a corneal infection and other problems with daily- or extended-wear soft contacts also increases. One study of 5,600 patients found that only 2 percent still had enough refractive error after one year to justify wearing contact lenses. About 60 percent of those wore rigid or gas permeable lenses, and approximately 30 percent wore soft contact lenses.

Keep in mind that many people consider vision correction surgery because they have problems wearing contact lenses. If you are contact-lens-intolerant before refractive surgery, you will probably continue to find them uncomfortable after radial keratotomy.

Some RK contact lens wearers say that they feel as if a speck of dust is in their eye as the lens floats over the reshaped corneal curvature. Others complain of fluctuating vision when they remove their lenses.

Finding contact lenses that are comfortable after RK may require patience. If your eye doctor has extensive experience in fitting contacts after incisional surgery, your chances of achieving a good fit increase dramatically. Eye doctors are trained to fit lenses that are steeper in the center and flatter in the periphery. Following RK the shape of the eye is the opposite: flatter in the center and steeper in the periphery. Studying the computerized topographic maps of the new shape of the cornea, the eye doctor picks a trial lens for the patient's eye. After temporarily staining the eye with fluorescein, the physician can see how the lens floats on the surface. Depending on the person, highly gas-permeable rigid lenses with thin edges and a large diameter often provide the best fit after RK. There is about a 25 percent chance that the first trial lens won't be the best fit.

Referring to a study headed by R.F. Hofmann, M.D., Dr. George Waring, an RK expert, writes, "Fifty-six percent of patients were successfully fitted with rigid gas-permeable lenses [after RK]." (In this context, a fit is considered successful when the patient is able to wear lenses all the waking hours of the day.) "Patients fitted with a daily wear soft contact lens had only a 37 percent success rate at one year. Fitting of custom toric soft lenses had a success rate of 33 percent. The overall success rate was 41 percent. Dr. Hofmann reviewed the patients' preoperative history of contact lens success or failure. Of the eighteen patients who were contact lens failures preoperatively, thirteen (72 percent) were still contact lens failures after surgery. For all those patients who were contact lens successes before RK, the chance of success was only 50 percent after refractive keratotomy" (1992).

After astigmatic keratotomy, patients "had only an 18 percent success rate with all types of contact lens attempts. The most common reasons cited for failure were: variable vision, irritation, increased neovascularization (blood vessels infringing on the corneal incisions), and increased hyperopia" (Waring, 1992).

If you have been unable to wear contacts after radial keratotomy, you might wish to seek out a doctor who has fitted many RK patients. Obviously, a fitter who has seen thousands of RK patients should have better results than someone right out of school.

ASTIGMATIC KERATOTOMY

Refractive surgeons can correct mild myopic astigmatism with an operation related to RK called "astigmatic keratotomy" (AK), or "arcuate keratotomy." Using transverse incisions called "T-cuts," or "arcs," ophthalmologists can flatten the cornea's steepest meridian, which has the most power to bend light (see fig. 8). Such incisions are perpendicular to the cornea's most powerful axis. As with radial keratotomy, the greater the number, length, and depth of incisions, the greater the effect. AK results are less predictable than those following RK. In addition, astigmatic incisions stabilize slower than radial ones. Nevertheless, depending on whether the person has residual nearsightedness with astigmatism or farsightedness with astigmatism, AK occasionally is a better choice than LASIK to re-treat patients who want to fine-tune their original operation.

Doctors can attempt to correct regular astigmatism with either LASIK or astigmatic keratotomy (AK). A "coupling effect" occurs with both surgical techniques. Choosing the proper astigmatic treatment depends on whether patients are near- or farsighted. When correcting the cornea's "out-of-roundness," the choice is either to flatten the steepest curve or steepen the flattest curve (see fig. 17). If the eye is both nearsighted and astigmatic, the doctor may want to use the laser to treat both problems at the same time. In other words, the laser flattens not only the steepest meridian but also steepens the flattest one. This coupling effect can induce more correction of the myopia than simply treating the astigmatism by itself. On the other hand, if the astigmatism comes with farsightedness, the surgeon may wish to correct both of these refractive errors at the same time with astigmatic T-cuts. With AK, the flat meridian steepens as the steepest meridian flattens. This means that as the astigmatism is treated, the farsightedness is reduced.

CHAPTER TEN

CHOOSING THE RIGHT REFRACTIVE SURGERY FOR YOU: LASIK, PRK, OR RK

Eyes without speaking confess the secrets of the heart.

—St. Jerome

When considering refractive surgery, you deserve to have sufficient information to work effectively with your doctor to choose the operation that's best. At this point, you may still have some doubt about which refractive procedure—LASIK, PRK, or RK, if any—might help you. The answer depends in part on your unique eyes, your glasses prescription, and your doctor's expertise. We have discussed each operation's specific advantages and disadvantages, including different potential side effects and complications. Now let's compare the three procedures, considering the general results for the varying degrees of refractive error, physiological effects on the eye, comfort of the patient, speed of visual recovery, and stability of results. We will also consider how operative techniques and costs influence doctors.

Without doubt, LASIK is currently the procedure of choice among most high-volume refractive surgeons. Since LASIK involves more surgical skill than PRK, eye doctors at first were hesitant to use LASIK except for severe myopia. Today, however, more and more experts recommend LASIK over the other refractive surgeries for almost all ranges of nearsightedness. Moreover, most informed patients are requesting this newer excimer laser procedure. After researching the subject, eye doctors from all over the world have asked us to perform LASIK on their eyes, but we have never had a single ophthalmologist or optometrist request PRK.

LASIK is usually the obvious choice for mild, moderate, and severe nearsightedness—even though the results for *low* myopia one year after surgery are about the same with all three operations. We usually recommend LASIK for astigmatism. Currently, hyperopic LASIK is the only surgical procedure available for farsightedness, although new techniques are being studied. Depending on the patient's refraction, however, we occasionally treat low amounts of this refractive error with astigmatic keratotomy (AK) (see fig. 8).

If you have -3 diopters of nearsightedness, your chances of getting 20/40 or better uncorrected visual acuity are about the same with LASIK, PRK, or RK—*if* the surgeon is about equally skilled in all three operations. Your recovery with LASIK, however, would be easier. In addition, after LASIK, your vision should be largely restored within days while, after PRK, the process may take months. With rare exceptions, if you have moderate or severe nearsightedness, we would suggest LASIK over PRK or RK. Although PRK results are improving with the new scanning lasers, as mentioned earlier, one large study showed that 13 percent of moderate and high myopic patients lost two or more lines of best-corrected visual acuity (BCVA) six months after PRK.

COMPARING THE PHYSIOLOGICAL EFFECTS ON THE EYE

You will recall that each surgical procedure has a unique physical effect on the eye. With RK the radial cuts in the mid-periphery of the cornea weaken the incised area. Each spoke-like incision made by the diamond-tipped knife cuts vertically through most of the stroma (the third, and middle, corneal layer), almost to Descemet's membrane, the fourth layer. This means that the incisions penetrate farther into the cornea than the excimer laser does. The more nearsighted the RK patient, the greater the number of incisions and generally the longer and deeper the slits. The normal pressure inside the eye causes tissue near the incisions to bend so that the sides of the cornea bow out, stretching and flattening the center. Necessary to correct nearsightedness, this weakening and bending effect is a drawback of RK surgery. If the cornea bends too much, the patient will become farsighted. If it bends too little, the person will be undercorrected.

Too much surgical treatment—too many incisions of too great a length—is needed to correct severe nearsightedness with RK. Since the RK wound-healing response of every person is different, doctors are unable to predict exactly how much surgery a person's cornea can sustain before it is weakened to the point that it becomes unstable. Although this RK complication is more prevalent in highly myopic patients, even a few people with low degrees of nearsightedness can develop fluctuating vision. Over time, some RK patients experience hyperopic shift, becoming farsighted. In addition, after radial keratotomy, diurnal changes in the pressure within the eye can cause fluctuating vision in some patients because the cornea moves or flexes. It is easy to see why this operation—which has helped many people see better—has technological limits.

After the RK incisions heal, they become fine scars that usually diminish somewhat over time. Since the central portion of the cornea remains uncut, patients seldom look through the incisions except when the pupil dilates. Nevertheless, this means that in dim light some RK patients complain of starbursts and glare, especially right after surgery.

Excimer laser surgeries have a totally different physiological effect on the eye from RK. Since the laser removes tissue at the sub-micron level, PRK and LASIK are much more precise than RK, which relies on the accuracy of a hand-held, diamond-tipped knife. All three procedures change the curvature of the cornea. PRK reshapes the corneal surface while LASIK sculpts the inner cornea, indirectly changing the eye's front curvature. LASIK patients look through a larger lens-like treated zone. They have no RK incision scars. Unlike RK, which slightly decreases the burst strength of the eye, neither laser-based procedure seems to weaken the cornea.

Comparing Patient Comfort

In the past, many eye doctors thought that PRK might be less traumatic than LASIK. PRK has no cutting phase or keratectomy and, after the gel-like covering is removed, only the cool laser light touches the corneal surface. The problem with PRK, however, is that when the protective epithelial layer is scraped away, the eye is left open and unprotected—exposed to the air during the initial healing process. To warn the brain that the eye is under attack, many of the pain fibers in the cornea are located near the surface. During the PRK treatment, the laser ablates right through this area. Until the debrided top epithelial layer grows back, the patient suffers from a painful corneal abrasion. Considering that during PRK the laser light exposes the nerve fibers, it is no surprise that, after the topical anesthetic wears off, patients can hurt.

A closer look at the physical effects of LASIK will help you further understand why LASIK is easier on people with all degrees of refractive error. A major advantage of surgery under a flap is that not only the first, but also the second, protective corneal layer is preserved—both the epithelium and Bowman's membrane remain almost totally intact. The epithelial layer seems to heal better if it can attach itself to Bowman's smooth surface, the second layer of the cornea that acts as a barrier against infection. During PRK, the laser cuts right through this membrane, partially or completely removing its central portion, leaving about one-third of the periphery untouched. The vaporized Bowman's tissue never grows back. With LASIK, Bowman's membrane, which helps protect the eye from insult, injury, and infection, is preserved because it is part of the flap.

Generally providing increased patient comfort and satisfaction, LASIK creates an optical zone, or newly-reshaped corneal "lens," that is larger than the RK clear zone. When the pupil dilates in dim light, some RK patients are aware of the fine spoke-like scars. Obviously, LASIK patients never have this problem.

From preceding chapters, you know that LASIK patients have minimal or no pain during and after surgery. As a rule, RK and PRK patients also almost never complain of pain during the actual procedure. Afterward, however, some RK patients must be treated for significant pain for a day or two. Following PRK, doctors unfortunately are unable to predict the amount of post-operative pain that people will experience: it can vary from slight to excruciating. After this surface surgery, patients often require strong oral analgesics while LASIK patients seldom fill their pain medication prescription.

In addition, with this newer laser procedure, the healing process occurs under the flap—away from the elements. The large surface abrasion following PRK hurts more than the edges of the LASIK flap. As a LASIK patient you would have an easier healing period with less tissue reaction. Of course, your ease of recovery after both laser operations also is related to the severity of your nearsightedness. The higher the degree of refractive error, the more tissue the excimer must remove and the greater the body's inflammatory response. This means that if you have moderate or severe myopia, LASIK is preferable to PRK.

During the immediate post-operative period, PRK patients need eye patches or bandage contact lenses. If you have LASIK, you would require eye drops for only about five days and the protection of a clear plastic shield for three nights only while you sleep. Your eye should look and feel almost normal the day after surgery or earlier.

COMPARING SPEED OF VISUAL RECOVERY

As mentioned throughout this book, LASIK patients have more rapid visual recovery than those who have PRK. RK patients also generally get their results rather quickly, often returning to work a few days after surgery. PRK has more temporary side effects related to the healing process that can slow recovery. Most LASIK patients see fairly well one to four days post-op, while PRK patients may take one to four weeks or longer to attain reasonably functional eyesight. (Older, highly myopic LASIK patients, even those with surgically induced monovision, may require several months to achieve their final near vision.)

PRK patients sometimes have corneal haze that looks like white, star-filled nebulae under the slit-lamp microscope, while LASIK patients seldom complain of this problem. Even though their corneas are clear, however, LASIK patients sometimes describe their vision as "hazy" immediately after surgery because their surgical correction is slightly inaccurate. Such hazy vision following LASIK is almost *never* caused by the type of physical corneal haze that is sometimes evident on microscopic examination after PRK. Fortunately, today's newest scanning lasers and advanced ablation techniques have significantly diminished the scarring associated with haze. Nonetheless, since the laser treatment of myopia occurs directly over the visual axis, or line-of-sight, PRK-induced haze can affect vision. Following PRK for moderate or severe myopia or for astigmatic treatments greater than -3 diopters, clinically significant haze can persist for weeks or even months. This problem, which seldom occurs with low myopia, may require lengthy treatment with steroid eye drops and many visits to the doctor. Some PRK patients need topical steroids for four months or longer while LASIK patients use this medication for less than a week. Sometimes, repeat surgery is required to reduce unresolved haze associated with PRK. All things considered, PRK has a higher risk of wound-healing complications than LASIK.

According to Louis E. Probst, M.D., and Jeffery J. Machat, M.D., in *LASIK: Principles and Techniques,* "The number of LASIK operations performed throughout the world continues to increase exponentially because of the advantages this procedure offers over PRK. While PRK involves a slow return of visual function, with poor vision during the epithelial healing for the first three or four post-operative days and a slow improvement of vision over the first month, LASIK often results in a dramatic visual improvement even by the first post-operative day and full visual recovery by three or four days post-operatively."

COMPARING STABILITY OF RESULTS

You are more likely to have stable results with LASIK than after RK or PRK. Unfortunately, over time some RK patients become farsighted—even though four-cut mini-RK with shorter incisions for low myopia has reduced hyperopic creep. Following PRK, doctors are unable to predict the amount of myopic regression that might occur in moderately and severely nearsighted patients. Such regression is seldom a problem with radial keratotomy because incisionally treated corneas tend to become flatter over time. Nevertheless, even RK patients can get more near-sighted if their eyeballs elongate. With LASIK, after a short recovery period, most people attain a fairly stable refraction. Some highly myopic persons, however, may experience moderate regression over time if their corneas steepen. Following both laser procedures, the middle layer of the cornea remodels itself where the laser removed tissue.

When PRK is performed for higher amounts of myopia, the epithelium may grow back thicker than after LASIK. Steepening the corneal curvature, this added epithelial thickness can nullify some of the beneficial effect of the surgery, causing the patient to regress. Of course, if the eyeball naturally becomes longer, myopia will get worse. Unfortunately, some severely nearsighted people have a tendency to become more myopic over time. Doctors are unable to prevent this natural progression. By topographically measuring the curvature of the cornea, doctors can tell if patients have corneal regression or progressive nearsightedness.

For months after LASIK, your surgeon could re-treat your eye by merely lifting the protective corneal flap. I often use LASIK to retouch undercorrected LASIK or PRK patients. I never use PRK to re-treat or enhance an original PRK operation because we don't know how thick the epithelium has grown back.

When we first started introducing LASIK into our practice under FDA-approved clinical trials, we had both PRK and LASIK patients sitting in our waiting room. The morning after surgery, the PRK patients definitely knew that something had happened to their corneas. After the procedure on their first eye, people would discuss their operations in detail. The PRK patients could see that the LASIK patients were much more comfortable and had better vision. The PRK patients would say, "My vision is blurry, and my eye hurts." The LASIK patients replied, "It hardly hurts at all, and I can see pretty well." When the PRK patients came back to have their second eye done, almost all of them said, "I want the other refractive surgery—the one called LASIK."

The relative simplicity of learning the PRK technique may make it attractive to ophthalmologists, but LASIK is what patients expect of refractive surgery.

RARE EXCEPTIONS

There are only a couple of medical situations in which we would choose PRK over LASIK. If you have scarring in the superficial layers of the cornea, we might recommend PRK. Since it is a surface procedure, the laser will remove damaged tissue on the front of the cornea. If you have an extremely poor epithelium, or if it is loose, we might pick PRK to avoid passing the keratome over a compromised eye. Some people have an unusually small or deep-set eye or a large brow. In such cases, the doctor might be unable to fit the LASIK suction ring on the eye. In these rare cases, we would recommend PRK instead of LASIK because it might be mechanically impossible to do the keratectomy to create the flap. Although we have a special technique for getting the suction ring on small eyes, in a few cases, the person's orbital anatomy precludes LASIK.

IN SUMMARY

Since LASIK provides more rapid return to vision—with much less discomfort than PRK—why are some eye doctors still doing the older operation? One reason is that after extensive clinical trials, PRK has been approved by the FDA while LASIK is simply permitted as a practice of medicine. PRK also is less expensive and technically demanding for the ophthalmologist to learn than LASIK. PRK requires a less thorough patient workup. The actual

PRK operation is not only much simpler to perform, it is less stressful for the surgeon. After entering the correction into the laser's computer and removing the epithelium, the PRK surgeon merely focuses the light scalpel over the eye's line-of-sight and lets the computer sculpt the corneal surface. The newer scanning lasers have reduced the incidence of surgical errors such as decentered laser treatments for both PRK and LASIK.

A far more demanding operation for the doctor, LASIK requires much more attention to detail. Good clinical judgment and precise surgical timing are important to excellent LASIK results. Every minuscule step is critical. Notwithstanding, as doctors observe firsthand the reduced recovery period following LASIK, they are switching to this newer operation. In the long run, LASIK saves both eye doctors and patients hours of follow-up time—no small advantage to all involved.

The surgical skill of the doctor is an important factor determining whether you might attain better results with LASIK, PRK, or RK. If you are under the care of an experienced LASIK surgeon, this procedure usually is the best choice. For someone in the hands of an ophthalmologist who has a limited knowledge of LASIK, PRK is the best choice. To dramatize the surgical nature of LASIK, surgeons sometimes say that the PRK procedure is 90 percent laser and 10 percent surgical skill while LASIK is 10 percent laser and 90 percent operative technique. So if we were planning to allow an inexperienced LASIK surgeon to operate on our eyes—which many patients do—we would prefer that he perform PRK rather than LASIK. As we emphasized earlier, LASIK has a steeper surgical learning curve than PRK because the protective flap must be carefully managed. For this reason, for the beginning refractive surgeon, PRK is a safer technique. Nevertheless, as increasing numbers of informed patients demand the more patient-friendly procedure, surgeons all around the world are learning LASIK. With intensive study and practice, this surgical technique is well within the skill level of corneal surgeons and many other ophthalmologists.

Many vision correction centers that only do PRK are closing their doors. No matter how much refractive surgeons advertise, they cannot stay in business without satisfied patients telling people about good results achieved with minimal disruption to their lives. Even though some PRK patients report excellent outcomes, they seldom recommend PRK to other people. Without such patient referrals, clinics lack the volume to cover their costs. In contrast, LASIK patients often recommend it to others—sending their friends and relatives from all over the U.S. and abroad to their doctors.

With any elective operation, the cost is always a factor. At some clinics, RK is cheaper than PRK or LASIK because, as mentioned earlier, the laser-based procedures require technologically advanced equipment that is expensive to maintain. To keep current with both surgeries, the doctor should update the laser if the newer models offer patients noticeably improved results. LASIK also is more costly to perform because of the high overhead associated with the surgical instrument that cuts the flap. The microkeratome costs tens of thousands of dollars and must be perfectly maintained. Entire chapters of refractive surgery books for eye doctors are devoted to this subject. Since safer, better keratome models have recently been developed, clinics incur additional expense when they upgrade this surgical equipment. The training of the LASIK surgeon is longer, more rigorous, and more expensive than the PRK surgeon. The question to keep in mind is: Should you shop for the cheapest operation when your future vision depends on the outcome? We don't think so. A better alternative might be to save your money until you can afford the best procedure for your eyes.

As one young, moderately nearsighted patient asked, "What's your opinion? Should I have LASIK or PRK? I like the idea that PRK involves less cutting. I want to see well. I want excellent results. But that's not all I want—I don't want the surgery to hurt. I want to get my results quickly. I want my outcome to be permanent. Since I am paid on commission, I can only miss one day of work. I can't spend much time at follow-up visits. And..." she added with a grin, "I want you to do the operation for free."

We explained, "LASIK is a more complicated operation than PRK. Nevertheless, LASIK meets more of your qualifications, although neither procedure can promise perfect results. When we first started doing PRK, we had high hopes for this surgical technique. But this operation can hurt like crazy for the first few days, especially since you have dry eyes. After PRK, you probably would have to take pain medications and wear bandage contact lenses. You might need steroid drops for months. You would have to make many visits to our clinic. In short, you will be inconvenienced if you have PRK."

For all the above reasons, we recommend LASIK over PRK in almost all cases, but especially if the myopic correction is in the higher ranges. As stressed earlier, doctors have learned to avoid treating extremely nearsighted people with RK. With the advent of the excimer laser, RK is almost an outdated operation except for correcting minor amounts of nearsightedness and astigmatism. Although most informed patients request LASIK, occasionally we have someone who absolutely insists on PRK—even after hearing all the facts. Perhaps the person is bothered by the idea of the LASIK keratectomy. Or perhaps she has a friend who now has normal 20/20 visual acuity after PRK. If she has -2 diopters or less of myopia, she has more surgical options than other people. Although this person might get about the same visual result with PRK, or even RK, as with LASIK, the physical effects on the cornea are considerably different.

After reading this chapter, you should be better able to weigh your doctor's advice. In the end, you alone—after consulting with your personal physician—can decide which operation, if any, might be appropriate for you. Only after thoughtful consideration can you pursue the goal of improved vision with reasonable assurance that you have made the best decision for your unique eyes and lifestyle.

CHAPTER ELEVEN

ENHANCEMENT: CAN YOU HAVE REFRACTIVE SURGERY AGAIN?

> *As the degree of myopia increases, so does the amount*
> *of regression from the initial myopic correction and the*
> *subsequent need for enhancement procedures.*
> —Louis E. Probst, M.D., and Jeffery J. Machat, M.D.
> *LASIK: Principles and Techniques*

Your mind flashes back to your sixth grade math class. Your teacher, Miss Andersen, is writing something on the blackboard. Since you have no glasses or contact lenses, you cannot see the story problem.

"What is the answer?" asks Miss Andersen. She is calling on you.

"I can't see the board," you reply softly, without raising your eyes.

"Well, why didn't you say so earlier? Bring your desk to the front of the room this instant," she says. Having perfect vision, she fails to understand why you are so shy about admitting that you cannot see.

Dragging your chair behind you, you put it right up against the blackboard. At first you don't notice, but your books, assignments, and pencils have left a paper trail all the way to the back of the room. The class giggles. In order to see where the pencils have rolled, you are reduced to crawling around on your knees with one hand holding your short skirt and the other searching for your things. The snickers grow louder.

At last, with your papers crumpled in one hand, you creep into your chair. "Well," says the teacher, certain that you finally can see the board, "I am waiting for an answer."

The problem is you still can't see the question. Feeling like Miss Magoo, you sheepishly get up and literally put your nose on the blackboard. Your classmates are now rolling in the aisles.

Far worse than Miss Andersen's math class was the sixth grade dance. You can remember your uneasy, prepubescent self, all arms and legs, sitting at the edge of the dance floor—totally alone. Your grandmother has pinned your waist-length hair into an old-lady's bun "to show off your ears"—as if they were important. Looking through your new, black spectacles—you sense that the rims look like horns pointing to the gym ceiling—you see your anxious parents standing by the door. You turn away quickly and spot your swimming buddy. Unable to see your eyes, he doesn't understand that you are looking at him. Like some impenetrable barrier, your glasses separate you from all the dancers. Not one classmate—not even your best girlfriend—appears to notice the yearning in your huge, liquid brown eyes.

You recall how, by age fifteen, puberty and contact lenses had totally changed your life. Now, twenty-two years later, you are back in glasses again, and they are "thicker" than ever.

Jackie

After suffering from years of disconcerting incidents caused by poor vision, you had hoped that a refractive eye operation would be the complete answer to all your prayers. At first, you probably were thrilled with the dramatic improvement. Perhaps your original operation greatly diminished your refractive error. But after the initial exhilaration, you might now feel a little let down because your vision is slightly less than perfect. The more nearsighted you were before your first procedure, the more likely you are to want additional surgery. If you still have to wear thin glasses part of the time, can another outpatient operation to fine-tune your eyesight get you closer to 20/40 or better?

Said one man, age thirty-seven, whom we corrected from -6 diopters to 20/40 without glasses: "I want to have an enhancement procedure to fine-tune my vision. When I first had this surgery, I marveled that I could finally see without glasses. But after a while, I got really angry. At last I could see the glint of light striking the edges of my cocktail table, but I wanted to see the fine dust under the four-legged teapot. I know you never promised me 20/20, but why stop short of perfect? I want my vision to be as good as it can be." Re-treatment brought his visual acuity to 20/25, or almost normal.

Your doctor might reoperate to enhance your vision if you are slightly unhappy with your original surgical results. In accomplished hands, LASIK is an excellent way to fine-tune PRK, RK, or LASIK surgery. With repeat operations, however, vital additional factors come into play—and every case is different. As with your first operation, your vision might improve, but your results still may be less than perfect.

You might want an enhancement for several reasons. Perhaps your primary operation left you a little under- or overcorrected. More residual nearsightedness than planned is quickly apparent. Such an initial *under*correction can occur if your doctor—in trying to avoid making you farsighted—is too conservative in the amount of tissue removed. Initial undercorrections also can occur if the laser beam varies or if the calculations are based on a small sample of patient results. Moreover, some factors determining visual results, such as how you heal, are totally beyond a doctor's control.

As we have emphasized, if you are nearsighted, your eyes are at least in focus *somewhere*, but if you are *over*corrected, as you pass age forty or so, you eventually won't be in focus *anywhere*. Keeping this in mind, you doctor will valiantly strive to avoid *over*correcting you (making you farsighted) by targeting your result slightly on the nearsighted side. You'll recall that farsightedness is more difficult to treat than nearsightedness. Reoperations to correct hyperopia are less predictable and available than those to correct residual myopia. Fewer ophthalmologists are expert in performing hyperopic LASIK.

What if you become a little nearsighted again after your first operation because you regress slightly over time? Even though your first operation was right on target, you might eventually lose some of the effect of surgery, especially if you had high myopia. Some regression, which usually becomes evident within three months (or even longer with severe nearsightedness), is associated with the healing process. Furthermore, if your eyeball naturally continues to elongate, you will become more nearsighted, although your eyesight should be much better than if you had never had refractive surgery.

Your doctor walks a fine line when trying to decide if enhancement surgery will meet your expectations. He probably will consider reoperating if your visual acuity is worse than 20/40 without glasses—assuming that your eyes healed well after your first refractive surgery. If you had greater than -6 or -8 diopters of nearsightedness, you have a higher probability of needing another operation than patients with less myopia. Some severely nearsighted patients are undercorrected by -1 diopter or more. If your residual myopia is *less* than -1 diopter, however, your surgeon must think long and hard before plunging into an enhancement procedure. Even though your chances of attaining better vision during a refinement procedure may be good, the risks are much greater the second time around. Never forget that reoperations—like all surgeries—have risks. If you put yourself under a laser light scalpel, a diamond-tipped knife, or a keratome blade for the second time, you face the same complication possibilities that follow the original operation—and *additional* risks as well. Operating on the surgically treated eye is always more risky than treating a virgin eye.

With your first LASIK surgery, the benefit-to-risk ratio is greatly in your favor. If you are moderately nearsighted, you have a better-than-90-percent chance of being able to drive without glasses after your original laser procedure. Your risk of significant complications is extremely small—if your doctor is highly skilled, if she uses the safest equipment, and if you follow your post-surgical directions. (Obviously, a boxer's glove in the eye the day after surgery could dislodge the protective flap.)

With enhancement surgery, however, the scale is tipped less in your favor. The potential benefits are lower, and the risks are considerably higher than with a primary operation. In fact, the second time around there's a greater chance that your eyesight might get worse, not better. Even though many people achieve great post-enhancement vision, hindsight is not always 20/20 after repeat surgery.

THE WISDOM TO SAY "NO"

Your surgeon wants the best possible visual acuity for you, but there are times when she must have the wisdom to say "no" to more surgery. Enhancement surgery demands greater in-depth knowledge than a primary procedure. More pitfalls must be avoided. The surgical plan and operative technique are more specialized. As with any procedure, physicians go through a steep learning curve when they first perform reoperations. Hence, your ophthalmologist's experience is even more critical than with a primary procedure. Keen clinical judgment greatly increases the chances of attaining excellent results. Interestingly enough, the more re-treatments eye surgeons see, the more selective they become about performing reoperations. Since I have re-treated many referred patients who came to me with less-than-satisfactory enhancement results, I now firmly believe that eye doctors should tell patients before their first operation: "Our first shot is the best one. Yes, I may be able to reoperate, but the risk of complications is higher with repeat surgery. In fact, many problems that I see occur during a second or third operation."

Sometimes, the most technically oriented people think that a refinement operation can tweak their eyesight to perfection. John, a thirty-year-old electrical engineer, wanted an enhancement procedure for residual nearsightedness after laser surgery. He said, "Okay, Doc, let's plan this next operation. I had eight diopters of myopia. You did two hundred pulses with the laser. That reduced my refractive error by seven diopters. So let's see… that means, to hit the target, we only have to do 26.5 more pulses, and I'll be 20/20!"

"It just doesn't work like that, John," I replied. "Surgery on the human body is a little like cutting a cherry pie. How many times can you cut each remaining piece in half? As you know, the answer is an infinite number of times. Theoretically, you can get an unlimited number of halves. Similarly, if you are left with one diopter of residual nearsightedness after LASIK, we might be able to treat another half diopter, but we can never promise to eliminate all of your refractive error. With repeat surgery, the risks are higher and the rewards are lower. Even with the submicron precision of the excimer laser and the reduced inflammatory healing response following LASIK, we are unable to guarantee perfection."

What your surgeon says about enhancement procedures before your initial operation can give you clues about the extent of his understanding of refractive surgery. In our opinion, you may want to find another doctor if he says, "Don't worry. If we don't get you close to 20/20 the first time, we'll simply do the procedure again."

He might be able to reoperate successfully, but only by putting your original results at some risk.

Another statement that shows a lack of comprehensive knowledge of enhancement surgery: "If you need a little more treatment, we can just re-lift the flap the week after surgery."

At first glance, this statement doesn't sound unreasonable. Re-lifting the corneal flap is certainly an early option. But, in truth, your physician won't know your exact outcome for at least three months. Your results might not be totally stable within a week, especially if you have high myopia. It makes no sense to remove more corneal tissue until the eye settles down because you might end up overcorrected. If your doctor waits a few months, additional surgery might be unnecessary.

It is the patient's responsibility—as well as the doctor's—to know when to walk away. One thirty-five-year-old banker said, "Wait a minute. Let me consider all the facts here: the first operation really improved my vision. It made me a lot better. LASIK didn't hurt. I had the surgery on Friday and drove to work on Monday. You're not going to charge me for an enhancement. It's free. Why not have it done again? There's nothing to lose."

But there is! We see referred enhancement patients who would give anything to recover the vision that they had after their first operation. One wealthy cardiologist said, "I'd pay two hundred thousand dollars to have the eyesight I had following my original LASIK procedure." Even though repeat surgery is usually performed at minimal additional monetary cost, there is definitely a time when you should say, "Let's call it quits, Doctor."

The point is that LASIK enhancement surgery sounds easy, but there is much less margin for error with a second operation. When contemplating your re-treatment, your doctor is thinking: her cornea is thinner, and it has been cut. Her refractive error is much less, so her vision will only be a little better. I have a much greater chance of making her farsighted. The second time around, she has a significantly increased risk of irregular healing. What are my chances of attaining a result that will make this patient happy?

REFINEMENT TECHNIQUES

There are several ways to re-treat a LASIK patient. During the first few months after the original operation, your surgeon can usually re-lift the flap. This sometimes is the safest enhancement technique. Loosening the gel-like epithelium at the upper edge of the flap, your doctor injects saline under the tissue and carefully re-lifts it. If the flap sticks in places, the doctor gently performs a lamellar resection, carefully freeing the adhered tissue. Gently raising the flap, he then applies a little more laser treatment to the corneal bed and repositions the flap—smoothing it out to avoid wrinkles. After this enhancement approach, the edge of the flap might not be as smooth as after the original operation. Hence, the eye doctor must vigilantly watch for epithelial ingrowth where the flap meets the stromal bed. Fortunately, this problem can usually be avoided with proper surgical technique. Some people experience post-operative discomfort for several hours after a refinement procedure.

If the protective flap has permanently re-attached to the corneal bed since the original LASIK operation, the surgeon must perform another keratectomy. After six months, re-lifting the flap becomes more difficult. Trained to operate within the corneal layers, high-volume refractive surgeons perform repeat surgeries on a daily basis—usually with excellent results. Nevertheless, once you understand the physiological effects of multiple parallel surgical cuts on the eye, you will see why the risk of complications is higher with any repeat procedure. After the first pass of the microkeratome blade, you are in effect looking through two nearly perfectly matched "plates of glass," so to speak. Where the surface of the protective flap and the middle corneal layer meet is one interface. Although you should be *totally* unaware of any reduction in visual acuity, an extremely *slight* subclinical degradation of the quality of vision can occur as the light passes through the interface.

With the second keratectomy, or surgical cutting of the flap, however, you are looking through "three plates of glass." Most enhancement patients are not aware of this effect either. They are usually thrilled with their results. Nevertheless, if the double interface is prominent, people can develop irregular astigmatism, leading to a noticeable reduction in the quality of their eyesight. A few persons have lost lines of best-corrected visual acuity on the eye chart after two operations.

No matter how good the doctor's motives, if the results are below par, everybody loses: the doctor because he literally puts his life's work on the line every time he picks up the keratome; but even more important, the patient because he may lose some of the benefits of the original vision correction surgery. Since I am willing to treat difficult cases, I often operate on referred patients who are unhappy with their enhancement results. A third operation to refocus the eye is not only riskier for patients but also extremely inconvenient.

REFINEMENT COMPLICATIONS

Perhaps the patient had requested the second procedure to diminish residual nearsightedness or astigmatism. But, unfortunately, the enhancement overcorrected her, and she became farsighted. As she approaches forty, she will become exceedingly unhappy with her eyesight. Once the crystalline lens inside the eye can no longer accommodate for farsightedness, she will be unable to see well not only in the distance but also up close. Even though glasses or contact lenses will focus her vision, the original goal of the refractive surgery was to make her less dependent on these optical crutches.

With the advent of hyperopic LASIK, we can now treat surgically induced farsightedness, whether the overcorrection follows a primary or an enhancement procedure. Refinement surgery for hyperopia is somewhat less accurate than a reoperation for myopia, but most patients are happy with their results—even if they achieve only a partial improvement. For older patients, any improvement helps at all distances. Younger people, of course, can compensate for some farsightedness. In any event, we sometimes recommend that people with a mild overcorrection delay having yet another surgery for up to a year because some persons gradually become slightly myopic again with time. In other words, they might regress enough to avoid more surgery. During this time, some older farsighted patients must wear glasses or contact lenses to focus well at any distance.

Another possible enhancement complication is irregular astigmatism, which is caused by a fine wrinkling of the protective flap's tissue or an unevenly ablated corneal bed. Highly experienced refractive surgeons are skilled at avoiding this problem, which is currently difficult to treat—even with the most advanced flying-spot lasers. To explain why the risk of irregular astigmatism increases with reoperations, Dr. Baker compares the surgical management of the protective flap to handling cellophane. If you are reasonably adept, the first time you touch it, you can create a smooth transparent surface. If, however, you fiddle with the tissue-thin wrap too much, you risk wrinkling it. A surgeon re-lifting the corneal flap must not only reposition it expeditiously but must also carefully control the tissue's hydration. Enhancement patients who develop irregular astigmatism must wear rigid contacts in order to see well. The new custom wavefront LASIK now under study may allow doctors to treat this complication with more success.

If Only We Had a Magic Wand

Mabel, a master chef and owner of a popular restaurant, returned to our office to ask if she could have an enhancement procedure. A forty-one-year-old grandmother, she carried one of her beautiful twin granddaughters in an infant carrier tucked under one arm. The baby was waving her tiny arms and grinning at us from under her pink lace bonnet. Mabel's daughter held the other child. Cuddled on her mother's shoulder, the little girl was rosy with sleep.

A strong-willed, red-headed woman, Mabel had LASIK three months earlier. Before her surgery, she complained that her glasses fogged up with steam when she cooked. Without them, she had been unable to read any letters on the eye chart. Now, after LASIK, her uncorrected visual acuity with both eyes was 20/30. Her corrected vision with glasses was 20/15—better than normal.

Mabel was absolutely determined to have a repeat operation on her *right* eye to focus it closer to 20/20 in the distance without glasses. After her original surgery, her dominant right eye had healed undercorrected by -0.75 diopters. I had purposely undercorrected her non-dominant eye by -0.75 diopters, which she planned to use for reading.

"I want you to correct my right eye another quarter diopter," Mabel told me. "I wore the trial contact lens for two weeks. It corrected my eye one-half diopter, but I've decided that a little less power would be better."

"I understand that you want to see better," I replied, "but I can't promise to treat only one-quarter diopter of nearsightedness."

"But, I have trouble with definition. I would like the letters to have more contrast—to be darker."

"The smallest increment of correction that we typically do with the laser is one-half diopter," I said. "We would never want to give you the misconception that LASIK is refineable to a quarter of a diopter."

"Well," she insisted, "let's do one-half diopter then. I am three-quarters undercorrected so that should leave me only one-quarter of a diopter nearsighted in my right eye. I'm not perfectly focused for the distance. My vision is a little hazy."

"Mabel," I replied, "surgery is just not that precise. We can aim for one-half diopter, but we may not get it. We cannot predict exactly how you will heal. Why don't you think about this for a few minutes while I see another patient. Dr. Baker also wants to talk with you."

"I hear that you aren't completely happy with your vision," Dr. Baker said.

"I see pretty well, but I want an enhancement operation on one eye. Dr. Slade doesn't seem to want to do more surgery on my eye. Did I say something wrong to him?"

"No, Mabel, I'm sure it's nothing you said. He just wants to make you happy—both now and in the future. Unfortunately, we cannot promise to get your vision exactly like you want it. If we reduce any more of your nearsightedness in your dominant eye, your close vision in that eye will get worse. As you get older, you will need magnifying glasses to read and to cook. Most of the time, you probably don't look in the distance."

"I will use my other eye to read," Mabel said, frowning.

"We certainly empathize with your desire for better distance vision. But even if we target your vision at a quarter-diopter of myopia, there is a chance that you might become farsighted, depending on how you heal. Over age forty, a little nearsightedness is preferable to even the slightest amount of farsightedness. If you are nearsighted, you are at least in focus *somewhere*. If you are overcorrected and become farsighted after your enhancement procedure, eventually, as you grow older, you won't be in focus in that eye *anywhere*."

"I understand," Mabel repeated, "but—as I *just* said—I will use my other eye for my close vision. I have thought about it for several months, and I am absolutely certain that I want an enhancement procedure. I will be *really* displeased if you refuse to do it!"

"We totally understand your motives. But unfortunately, if you become farsighted, you will have to wear a contact lens in that eye to see *at any distance* once your crystalline lens inside your eye can no longer compensate. At present, would you wear a contact lens in your dominant eye more than 50 percent of the time, or can you get along without correction most of the day?"

"If you won't do an enhancement, I will have to wear a contact lens in my right eye every hour that I'm awake. You are supposed to reoperate for free. But if Dr. Slade won't help me, I will find another doctor to do my enhancement—even if I have to pay an additional two grand," Mabel said angrily.

"Well, let me talk this over with Dr. Slade. I don't know if he'll do more surgery to treat such a small refractive error. He almost *never* does a keratectomy to re-treat only one-half diopter, but maybe he can re-lift the flap. When we test people's eyes, there is typically about a three-quarter diopter depth of focus where most folks can't tell the difference between the power of the lenses. In other words, if I ask patients: 'Which is better—one or two?' many people can't tell which power is stronger. So the question is: Is it worth risking more surgery for such a small change?"

"Well, *I* can tell the difference. So try to convince him," Mabel said. "I have thought about it a lot, and I know what I want! If I don't have an enhancement procedure, I will have to wear a contact lens in my right eye for distance. Yes, I know that after another operation, I might still have to wear one contact, but I also have a good chance of getting rid of it. I hate glasses, and contacts bother me because my eyes are extremely dry."

"Are you are saying that you are willing to accept the slight risk that you might get worse—in other words, become farsighted—after your second operation because you will have to wear a contact anyway?"

"Yes."

"If you had said that you get along without lenses over 50 percent of the time, I would have asked if you realize that you might lose all those lens-free times if you have additional surgery. In other words, if you get worse, you would be forced to wear correction, whereas without further surgery, you wouldn't need a contact much of the time. In this case, you would be functioning most of your life without corrective lenses. Why would you want to risk that?"

"But I *will* need one contact if I don't have another operation," Mabel insisted.

"I see. Let me get Dr. Slade," Dr. Baker said.

Returning to her examining room, I told Mabel, "I can try to treat another half diopter of your nearsightedness. Is that what you want?"

"Yes. That is *exactly* what I want. Can you do it right now so I can go home? My daughter is sitting in the waiting room with my twin grandbabies. Did you see them?"

"Yes, Mabel. They're cute."

"Thanks. They are a handful," Mabel said, proudly.

"You know that we are talking about the vision that you will have for the rest of your life?"

"Yes. I want to live my life with the best eyesight possible."

"I'll do an enhancement for you. Any time you have surgery, there are risks. I'll make every effort to avoid overcorrecting you, but I cannot predict how you will heal. If you become farsighted, you will require contacts lenses or glasses again. In other words, there is some risk that your vision might get worse—not better."

"I understand," said Mabel.

"Any time we do an enhancement operation," I said, "the risks are higher than with the first surgery, and the benefits are less—in your case, they are *much* less. The risk of infection, though *extremely* rare, is always with us. The probability that something might go wrong is higher with reoperations. Complications *do* happen. Some of them we can't repair."

"I know," Mabel said. "I have read the informed consent—twice."

"All right, Mabel. We are in this together," I said.

Mabel's Reoperation

Examining Mabel's eye under slit-lamp magnification, I marked the flap's edge. Then my surgical technician helped Mabel lie down under the laser. Looking through the operating microscope, I carefully—and I do mean *carefully*—lifted the original flap. Since she was only three months post-op, another keratectomy was unnecessary. After about a half-year, lifting the flap becomes increasingly more difficult, although every patient heals a little differently. I had preprogrammed the laser to remove a minimal amount of corneal tissue. Trying to reduce her myopia by 0.5 diopters, I performed her second procedure. After the treatment, I repositioned the flap and checked that it was properly aligned. It had adhered to the corneal bed.

At her follow-up visit the day after surgery, Mabel's unaided visual acuity had improved ever so slightly. We never saw her again. She is under the care of her regular eye doctor. We assume that she is satisfied with her results because we almost always hear immediately if a patient has problems.

We would love to have a magic wand that could correct vision to -0.25 diopters with no risk to the quality of the images falling on the retina. While the goal is to have patients walk out of the office happy, even using today's razzle-dazzle technology, there are limits to what we can do. Patients often have a long list of reasons for requesting a second operation. We never discount the need for better vision, but we also have to try to protect the improvement patients have after their original surgery—to protect their original investment. With the first operation, there is little risk that a patient's eyesight might get worse—if the procedure is done properly. With an enhancement operation, however, we always have to warn people that there is a slightly greater chance of degrading their best-corrected visual acuity (their vision *with* glasses) than with the original procedure. This risk should never be discounted—it is real.

Mabel knew what she wanted—and she got it. She would have been unhappy if we had refused to fine-tune her vision. In her case, since I have performed thousands of LASIK operations, I believed that the odds were in our favor. Nevertheless, -0.75 diopters of residual nearsightedness is a borderline case. If she had been -0.5 diopters undercorrected, I probably would not have performed an enhancement operation for her.

Mabel's case is the exception. We almost never perform repeat LASIK to enhance such a small refractive error—no matter how much a patient pressures us for more surgery. Why? What if Mabel's vision in her dominant eye *without* glasses had improved to -0.25 diopters, but her eyesight with glasses had dropped from perfect to 20/40? Would the enhancement procedure have been justified? We think not. As Mabel's doctors, it was our job not only to attempt to refine her uncorrected distance vision but also to preserve her best-corrected visual acuity. Until Mabel experiences the increasing effects of presbyopia that come with age, she won't understand the value of being a little nearsighted in her non-dominant eye. Looking ahead, refractive surgeons must try to anticipate their patients' future vision problems while meeting their current expectations.

It is really disappointing to hit the targeted enhancement correction exactly on the mark and still have the patient dissatisfied. This can happen when the person doesn't understand presbyopia or aging eyes. A few years after surgery, one patient said, "I can see better out in the distance, but when I'm reading in bed now, I can't see as well as I used to."

"Well," I explained, "you were thirty-seven when you had your first refractive surgery, and now you're forty-two. Eyesight is not a static thing. Remember when we discussed how your near vision would blur as you age, especially if you are 20/20 in the distance in both eyes. None of us want to accept presbyopia. We all want to see at least as well as we did when we were twenty-five. But, so far, we don't know how to prevent the natural loss of the flexibility of the crystalline lens."

Your Pre-enhancement Evaluation

Before considering LASIK enhancement, your doctor will thoroughly review your first operation's details. Your refraction must be stable—with little change in your correction over the last months since your first surgery. Your physician will assess the transparency of your cornea with the slit-lamp microscope and carefully measure the remaining thickness of your residual corneal bed. To ensure a safe re-treatment, the supportive middle corneal layer must be thick enough to permit another operation. In addition, your doctor will study your pre- and post-operative corneal topographic maps. If more surgery seems advisable, they will help him plan your operation.

How soon a reoperation is possible depends on which type of refractive surgery you originally had. If you had LASIK, your doctor usually can perform an enhancement after a three-month waiting period, sometimes sooner. At this stage, much of the regression sometimes found in people with high myopia has occurred, and the surgeon can still lift the flap. In many cases, I perform a second keratectomy. I usually wait six to twelve months before re-treating after a primary PRK procedure. If you've had RK, the waiting period is one year to allow for the surgical refraction to stabilize.

CORNEAL TRANSPLANTS

Consider this worst-case scenario: a patient comes into our office with such a severely diseased or scarred cornea that she has lost vision. How can we help this woman? Sometimes I can remove superficial opacities using "phototherapeutic keratectomy" (PTK), a special excimer laser procedure. If the corneal scars are deep, however, the woman may be faced with a corneal transplant. It may take over a year to get her final results, but a transplant operation may eventually enable her to see again. Doctors refer to this micro-surgical procedure as either "lamellar" (also called "partial") or "penetrating keratoplasty," depending on whether *half* the depth or the *entire* thickness of the cornea is replaced. Eye surgeons perform about ten thousand transplants every year in the U.S. Since the cornea normally lacks blood vessels, the body's immune system that usually attacks donor tissue fails to get the message that the graft is foreign. For this reason, this serious operation enjoys a high success rate. Although rejection of the donated tissue can occur immediately after surgery or years later, the initial transplant is rejected in only about 5 percent of cases. In every instance, the patient must be carefully monitored for possible infections and rejection of the transplanted tissue. Immediate intervention by the doctor can often control such complications.

The ultimate goal of a corneal transplant is to create a clear, smooth, more normally shaped window for the eye. Then refractive surgery may help the person achieve a corneal curvature that puts an in-focus image on the retina. Using the excimer laser to remove the central portion of the patient's clouded cornea, the doctor places donated corneal tissue from a recently deceased person on the recipient's eye. As you might well imagine, a perfect fit, which is achieved by using the same-sized, "cookie-cutter" instrument to cut both corneas, is crucial to decrease post-surgical astigmatism. The surgeon must stitch the edges of the transplanted cornea into the recipient's eye so that the circular junction is water tight. There is traction where the donor cornea is attached to the recipient's eye. The taut sutures cause wrinkles in the cornea. This means that the person's initial vision may be poor. During the first six months, neither glasses nor contact lenses clearly correct the patient's vision.

Unfortunately, until the tension on the cornea lessens, the doctor is unable to correct the person's eyesight. Over time, as the sutures loosen, the tissue relaxes so that the folds in the cornea become smoother. Physicians have no way of knowing what the final curvature—and thus the focusing power—of the donor cornea will be after it is attached to the recipient's eye. The transplanted corneal curvature might be flatter or steeper than the patient's excised tissue. The human graft also sometimes is "out-of-round," causing astigmatism. The refractive power will be based on how tight or how loose the new tissue lens is stitched into the eye. In other words, theoretically, the surgeon could sew an identical corneal graft into two people, but the final curvature could be completely different for each person. One patient's refractive error might improve while another's might not. No one will know the final effective refractive power of the transplanted corneal lens until the 360-degree circular wound heals.

After a corneal transplant, almost all patients have some refractive error. Unfortunately, without vision correction surgery, the patient has to accept the effective power of the transplanted cornea. Totally beyond the control of the doctor, wound-healing can have a dramatic effect on the focusing ability of the new cornea. The eye may heal mildly or extremely nearsighted, farsighted, or astigmatic. In addition, most transplant patients have a different refractive error in each eye. So a year after surgery, the person may have a basically new, healthy, clear, smooth, regular cornea, but its power might be significantly different from the other eye. A severe imbalance between the two eyes is absolutely miserable for the patient. Worse yet, this person cannot tolerate glasses. Imagine looking through a strong -8 diopter glass lens with one eye and a weak -1 diopter lens with the other. You would be totally unbalanced when corrected with such spectacles because of the large difference in image size falling on each retina. Only contact lenses or vision correction surgery can help. Unfortunately, not everybody can wear contact lenses, which may be especially difficult to fit after a transplant operation.

LASIK does carry added risks after a transplant but, by bringing both eyes into balance, has transformed the lives of many patients. About a year after the transplant, when the new cornea is stable, we can use the laser either to try to balance the eyes or to reduce or eliminate their nearsightedness, farsightedness, or astigmatism. With LASIK we attempt to get the person totally out of glasses, but sometimes we only succeed in making the refractive power of the two eyes more alike so that the person can at least wear thinner glasses.

CHAPTER TWELVE

FINE-TUNING PRK AND RK

*Success is getting what you want. Happiness
is liking what you get.*

—H. Jackson Brown

FINE-TUNING PRK WITH LASIK

If you've had PRK, and the amount of refractive error is still unacceptable, can LASIK or more PRK further improve your visual acuity? Every case is different, but LASIK might be able to fine-tune your PRK result. Currently, I never re-treat PRK with more PRK. Of course, after the original laser surgery, the nearsighted cornea is always thinner, and the corneal surface topography has changed. The primary PRK operation temporarily removed the epithelium and lasered the second and third layers of the cornea. The epithelium may grow back thicker or thinner than it was originally, leaving the corneal lens either steeper or flatter than needed for proper focus. Hence, the second time around, when doctors remeasure the thickness of cornea, they are unable to determine exactly how much residual nearsightedness is caused by a laser undercorrection of the stroma and how much is induced by a thickened epithelium. If it grew back too thick the first time, what's to keep the gel-like coating from building up too much after a second operation? In our opinion, in most cases, it makes no sense to re-treat with PRK again.

A close look at LASIK and PRK enhancements quickly reveals why we only re-treat PRK with LASIK. Safely preserved within the LASIK flap, the epithelium over the line-of-sight is basically undisturbed. Since it doesn't have to "re-epithelialize," or cover a large PRK wound, epithelial regrowth has little effect on the refractive outcome of the surgery. After a LASIK re-treatment of a primary PRK procedure, the cornea has been exposed to only one pass of the automated microkeratome blade. Moreover, all the other advantages of LASIK over PRK apply with the second operation, including increased patient comfort, rapid visual recovery, and avoidance of long-term steroid use to combat corneal haze. But no matter how easy the re-treatment is on the patient, the compelling question to keep in mind is whether the benefits of another operation are worth the increased risk of side effects and complications.

ENHANCING RK WITH LASIK

If you've had RK and still have a significant refractive error—either near- or farsightedness—an expert *might* be able to fine-tune your vision with LASIK. Although this procedure is an excellent way to enhance an original RK operation, re-treating RK must always be approached with extreme caution. The tolerances for error are minuscule. Before you even consider an enhancement, your eyes will require at least a one-year healing period. You and your doctor can then discuss reoperating—if the integrity of the eye has been maintained, if it has healed normally, and if the cornea is healthy. He will look for any irregularity or abnormal scarring and for the slightest loss of best-corrected visual acuity from the primary procedure. Your physician must carefully assess the stability of your cornea and the quality of the RK incisions. Your eye chart readings should be about the same from month to month over a reasonable period. Currently, we never enhance RK with PRK. Nor do we reopen RK incisions or cut more of them to correct residual nearsightedness.

If a large amount of nearsightedness—greater than -6 diopters—was treated with your original RK operation, the cornea might be unstable. If your post-RK visual acuity fluctuates because the cornea flexes, the laser *cannot* make your cornea more stable. A LASIK enhancement can only refocus the eye so that your vision fluctuates around a more desirable number. In other words, LASIK might improve your post-RK refractive status, but your surgeon must inform you that he is "shooting at a moving target." To illustrate, let's say your eyesight currently vacillates 1 diopter on either side of -3.5 diopters. After an enhancement procedure with LASIK, your vision would still waver 1 diopter, but you should be focused closer to 20/20, or plano. That is to say, your visual acuity might fluctuate plus or minus 1 diopter, but closer to normal instead of around -3.5 diopters. You should have better functional vision, but it would still be unstable—even after a second operation.

Before an RK patient undergoes a LASIK enhancement, the incisions from the first surgery should be well healed: there must be no epithelium in the wall of the slits, and the wounds must have closed, becoming fine scars. As mentioned earlier, healing defects such as residual epithelium in the incisions were usually associated with the older metal blades or re-opened RK incisions. Obviously, doctors try to avoid running a microkeratome blade across a RK incision that still has epithelium in the wound. If epithelial cells are 160 microns below the surface, the blade could spread some of them between the surfaces. Without proper attention, the person can lose vision if the epithelial cells proliferate into the interface. In addition, the corneal flap created during a LASIK enhancement of RK must be handled with great skill because it consists of four to eight pie-like wedges held together by the epithelial membrane and scar tissue.

As covered in chapter 9 in detail, some RK patients had initial overcorrections, and some have experienced hyperopic creep over time—but either way, they end up farsighted. Today, doctors sometimes can treat this problem with hyperopic LASIK. The best enhancement results are achieved with small degrees of farsightedness; the worst with severe hyperopia (see chapter 2 to review details about hyperopic LASIK).

Chapter Thirteen

THE NEW EVER-CHANGING PERIPHERAL TECHNOLOGY

The mind has a thousand eyes, and the heart but one.
—Francis William Bourdillon

Vision correction surgery is constantly advancing as researchers all over the world seek better ways to improve eyesight. When extensive clinical trials indicate that a new innovative procedure is reasonably safe and effective, it may become part of mainstream medicine. Unfortunately, a few people with extremely severe refractive errors fall outside the practical range of laser surgery. Doctors must conscientiously strive to find solutions for these patients. It is almost impossible for a normally sighted or even a moderately nearsighted person to understand what it is like to wear extremely strong glasses. Such spectacles can restrict the visual field, create distortions and aberrations, and reduce night vision. Not all highly myopic and hyperopic patients are able to wear contact lenses. These individuals are the ones who need help the most. To inform people about the ever-changing peripheral technology, this chapter not only discusses some new, highly investigatory surgical techniques to diminish severe refractive errors, but also some developing treatments for all ranges of vision.

Eye doctors have long dreamed of a refractive procedure that would be reversible or one that at least could be modified as the patient's prescription changes. Although the term "reversible surgery" is an oxymoron, the idea is undeniably interesting. To this end, we will discuss a new operation recently approved by the FDA that has the potential to be alterable over time.

Cataract Surgery and Clear-Lens Replacement Surgery (Refractive Lensectomy)

If you are extremely nearsighted with a refractive error of greater than -12 to -14 diopters or are very farsighted with a correction greater than +5 diopters, your doctor probably cannot treat your eyes with LASIK. Are there any other medical procedures that can help? As always, the answer hinges on your age, your eyes, and your surgeon. Depending on the clarity of your crystalline lenses inside your eyes, your doctor may tell you about several operations under study that are technically rather similar to a cataract operation. The benefits must be carefully weighed against the risks of surgically entering the eye.

Of course, if you are severely nearsighted or farsighted and if you have a clinically significant cataract, your ophthalmologist may suggest replacing the clouded crystalline lens with an artificial intra-ocular lens (IOL). The implant should allow clearer light to reach your retina and also should have the power to correct all or part of your refractive error (see fig. 26). Medical insurance usually covers the cost.

A highly-sophisticated surgical technique that has restored sight to millions, cataract surgery is considered fairly safe—even though all operations carry risks. Considering the complexity of the procedure, modern cataract surgery is relatively easy on the

Removing the Cataract

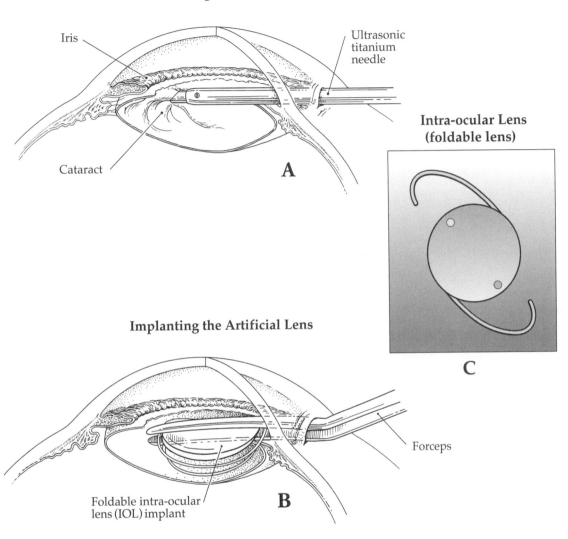

Iris

Ultrasonic
titanium
needle

Cataract

A

Intra-ocular Lens
(foldable lens)

C

Implanting the Artificial Lens

Forceps

Foldable intra-ocular
lens (IOL) implant

B

Figure 26

Cataract surgery using the "phacoemulsification" technique.

A. Removing the cataract or clouded crystalline lens from inside the eye. Holding a vibrating ultrasonic titanium needle, the surgeon breaks up the cataract and aspirates its fragments through a tiny hole in the instrument.

B. Implanting the artificial lens. Using miniature forceps, the microsurgeon slips an "intra-ocular lens" (IOL), or foldable artificial implant, inside the capsule that held the clouded crystalline lens.

C. The artificial intra-ocular lens that replaces the cataract or clouded natural lens.

patient. Some people go home and cook lunch the day after an operation. Nevertheless, whenever doctors operate inside the eye to take out the natural lens, they worry about the risk of infection, glaucoma, and retinal detachment. Generally, the more nearsighted the person, the greater the risk of retinal problems.

But what if you have no vision-impairing cataract, yet you cannot be comfortably corrected with any corrective lenses and your refractive error is beyond the help of LASIK, PRK, or RK? If you are old enough to have also lost much of your accommodative capability to see close, an operation called "refractive lensectomy," or "clear-lens replacement," might rehabilitate your distance vision. A few doctors will do this operation for older persons with refractive errors that fall outside the range of LASIK. As the name implies, during a clear-lens replacement, the surgeon removes the crystalline lens—which has no cataract—and replaces it with a refractive IOL. The goal is to diminish an *extreme* focusing error. Though performed in other countries, this surgery—which carries the risks of operating inside the eye—is still under study in the U.S. Considered an elective procedure, clear-lens replacement is not usually covered by insurance—no matter how disabled the patient.

One of the best ways to remove a crystalline lens—whether it has a cataract or not—is called "in-the-bag phacoemulsification" (see fig. 26). An amazing surgical technique, "phaco," as doctors refer to it—which is not laser-based—is a more delicate operation than brain surgery. Looking at the surgical field through a microscope, the cataract surgeon makes a tiny incision (about 3 millimeters wide) in the anesthetized cornea. An injection of a shock-absorbing liquid called a "viscoelastic" solution helps reduce the trauma to the intra-ocular tissues. To remove the crystalline lens, which sits behind the pupil and iris, the doctor must pass tiny instruments through the fluid-filled anterior chamber. It is under pressure. Rather as a grape has an outer skin, the clear lens (or clouded cataract) is surrounded by a capsule of tissue (see figs. 4 and 26). To reach the nucleus of the lens, the ophthalmologist must make a circular incision in this sac-like membrane. A tiny stream of pressurized water frees the nucleus from the outer portion of the lens known as the "cortex." Using a vibrating, ultrasonic titanium needle, the surgeon emulsifies, or breaks up, the nucleus and aspirates the fragments through a little hole in the instrument. Next, the doctor removes the cortex of the lens. Ideally, the remainder of the capsule stays in place. Holding miniature forceps, the surgeon gently slips a soft, foldable implant, or intra-ocular lens (IOL), inside the capsule that held the crystalline lens. Most of the viscoelastic solution is aspirated from the eye. A stitch to close the incision usually is unnecessary.

The IOL is designed to correct much of the person's near- or farsightedness, but as yet, the implant cannot compensate for astigmatism. Nevertheless, an ophthalmologist expert in refractive surgery can try to reduce the astigmatism by placing the corneal incision—the one used to enter the eye to remove the clouded lens—in the meridian of the cornea with the steepest curvature. In other words, rather like astigmatic keratotomy (AK), the corneal incision may reduce the astigmatism by flattening the steepest corneal axis. Although this clever surgical technique has helped many astig-matic patients, it seldom totally eliminates the problem. In some cases, I use laser surgery on the cornea to refine the remaining residual refractive error.

Remember, when people have their adjustable lens replaced, they lose their ability to accommodate—to see close without reading glasses. Of course, by the time most patients are old enough to need cataract surgery, their lens already has lost much of its ability to focus near objects. With clear-lens replacement surgery, however, even some older patients may still have some accommodative ability before the operation. With current lens replacement techniques, all such flexibility is lost. In the near future, doctors hope to have an implantable, flexible intra-ocular lens that actually moves with the eye to focus close objects.

It is easy to understand why clear-lens extraction to reduce severe refractive errors mimics cataract surgery. During a refractive lensectomy, the surgeon removes the crystalline lens—which has no cataract—and places an artificial IOL inside the capsule that held the clear natural lens. Selecting the power of the implant takes experience. It is a tricky calculation. Currently designed to improve mid-range and distance vision, IOLs—which potentially can provide good contrast sensitivity, or crisp vision—often can be fit to correct all of the near- or farsightedness.

Unfortunately, a few patients have such a high refractive error that even an IOL fails to provide adequate power. As with cataract surgery, the artificial lens currently fails to correct astigmatism. Hence, unless the cataract incision significantly reduces astigmatism, it must be corrected with glasses (or contact lenses if the patient can wear them). To restate for emphasis: as with cataract surgery, when the natural human lens is aspirated, the patient loses the ability to change focus to see close up. This means that lensectomy is seldom a good option for younger people—they obviously don't want to give up this accommodative ability. Nor do they want to wear reading glasses. Currently under study, a new implantable artificial lens that can change focus may allow some future lensectomy patients to read without magnifiers. As you might expect, clear-lens replacement and cataract surgery basically carry the same risks. Even though refractive lensectomy may successfully rehabilitate vision, any elective operation performed inside the eye requires a huge step emotionally for both the patient and surgeon.

MULTIFOCAL INTRA-OCULAR LENSES

Years ago, researchers tried to address the problem of presbyopia in older people by developing "multifocal intra-ocular lenses" that provide some depth of focus and reading vision after cataract surgery. Achieving limited success, these artificial lenses have varying refractive powers across the surface. This means that each incoming image is focused at several distances, including near and far. Presented with these multiple images, the brain has to sort out what it wants to see. For some people, this multifocal lens works fairly well; for others, the loss of fine detail, or "contrast sensitivity," which is exacerbated in dim light, is unacceptable.

SURGICAL TREATMENT OF PRESBYOPIA NOW UNDER STUDY

A new way of treating presbyopia, which is currently in clinical trials, attempts to provide accommodative ability in people needing reading glasses by implanting tiny plastic rods in the white outer-covering of the eye. The natural crystalline lens is not removed. To provide near vision, these rods stretch the outer circumference of the eye, partially restoring the ability of the inner muscles to change the shape of the lens. In a way, this procedure boosts the mechanical advantage of the muscles.

A FLEXIBLE ARTIFICIAL LENS TO FOCUS NEAR AND FAR

An exciting advancement in eye care, a new type of variable-focus intra-ocular lens should help reduce the need for reading glasses in cataract surgery patients. As covered throughout this book, before surgery, these folks have a clouded lens and presbyopia. Doctors have recently started replacing cataracts with a *flexible* artificial lens that can accommodate, or change shape, to focus close objects. Following this revolutionary technique, which may improve the daily lives of millions of older Americans, the eye will be able to refocus as it changes its gaze from far to near. I think that further study will prove that patients will have much of their near-focusing power restored following this procedure. In other words, after cataract surgery, many patients no longer will need bifocals because their new lens will change shape—becoming rounder as a young person's can. Achieving good results, I was privileged to per-form the first two such operations in the United States in March 2000. Of course, this procedure carries all the risks of cataract sur-gery such as infection, retinal detachment, and glaucoma.

The new lens-replacement procedure works because, as doctors have recently discovered, the muscles that are indirectly attached to the lens capsule can still move the lens in older people. Remember, the capsule surrounds the lens rather as skin covers a grape. For the patient to accommodate, surgeons must leave this capsule in place when they remove the partially hardened cataract. Keep in mind that the capsule is connected to the focusing muscle via tiny string-like zonular fibers. Since the new artificial lens is flexible, the mus-cles can move it so that the patient can see up close.

Doctors and researchers are working together diligently to pro-vide a solution to the problem of presbyopia.

REFRACTIVE INTRA-OCULAR LENSES (IOLS) OR IMPLANTABLE CONTACT LENSES (ICLS)

Some eye surgeons are correcting up to -18 diopters of extreme nearsightedness and +12 diopters of profound farsightedness with refractive "intra-ocular lenses" (IOLs), also called "implantable contact lenses" (ICLs). During this procedure, the surgeon implants an artificial lens inside the eye without removing the natural lens. The FDA is studying this operation in clinical trials for both effectiveness and safety in a carefully selected group of patients with moderate and severe near- or farsightedness.

There are several ways to place an ICL inside the eye. Some surgeons are putting the implant in the posterior chamber between the iris and the crystalline lens. When thus placed, the implant is called a PCIOL (a posterior chamber intra-ocular lens). Some doctors put an implant called an ACIOL (an anterior chamber intra-ocular lens) in the anterior chamber. Obviously, the ICL cannot find a home in the lens capsule because the natural lens remains in place.

A potential advantage of this surgery for a younger patient is that the person maintains the ability to focus up close because the natural clear crystalline lens is left in place. One disadvantage is that, in order to place the artificial lens within the eye, the doctor must operate inside the eye with all the concomitant risks, including infection, cataract formation, and glaucoma. Doctors also worry about the effect of the implant on the vital corneal endothelium. Other problems are possible. Continued improvements in ICL design are ongoing, and more studies are underway. Though they might be safer than removing the natural lens, an important question remains unanswered: What is the long-term safety of these devices?

"INTACS," OR "INTRA-STROMAL CORNEAL RING SEGMENTS" (ICRS)

"Intacs," or "intra-stromal corneal ring segments" (ICRS), are devices used in a new procedure to correct the lower ranges of nearsightedness (up to about -2 or -3 diopters). Following ICRS implantation surgery, which was approved by the FDA in 1999, some patients report high quality vision. Intacs are two tiny, plastic half-rings, or arcs, that together have the approximate diameter of a contact lens (see fig. 27). The rings are made of a biocompatible plastic used in cataract surgery. Inserted in tiny pockets in the anesthetized cornea during an outpatient procedure, the ring segments may correct myopia by flattening the curvature of the window of the nearsighted eye.

Intacs, or Intra-stromal Corneal Ring Segments (ICRS)

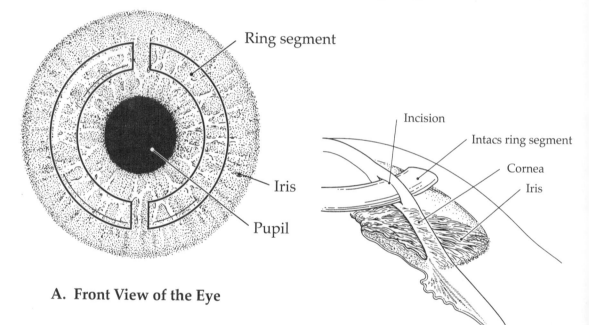

A. Front View of the Eye

B. Three-dimensional View of the Eye

Figure 27

"Intacs" or "Intra-stromal Corneal Ring Segments" (ICRS). A new procedure to correct mild nearsightedness.

A. Front view of the eye. Intacs, or corneal rings, are inserted in the periphery of the anesthetized cornea.

B. Three-dimensional view of the eye. Bending the eye's most powerful lens, the ring segment implants must remain in place in the middle layer of the cornea to reduce nearsightedness.

The effect of this operation is over the visual axis, or line-of-sight, but the incision and ring segments do not touch this area when they are positioned properly. Intacs are removable, with a high likelihood of reversibility of the refractive effect. This means that this procedure is adjustable—if the prescription changes or if the person is dissatisfied with the implant, it can be surgically removed. Always remember, however, that no surgery is truly reversible.

To insert intra-stromal corneal ring segments in the front of the eye, an ophthalmologist makes two tiny (about 2-millimeter) incisions in the periphery of the cornea. Slipping a special, curved dissection instrument into each incision, the doctor creates a tiny tunnel at a depth of two-thirds into the cornea. One covered channel runs along each side of the circumference of the window of the eye. A half-ring segment slides between the lamellar fibers in each respective side of the cornea. Bending the eye's most powerful lens, the device must remain in place in the middle, or stromal, layer of the cornea to achieve the effect.

U.S. studies have reported minimal side effects, although some patients have had peripheral haze, irregular healing, and other problems. According to Keravision, makers of Intacs, "Some patients experience difficulty with night vision, glare, halos, blurry or double vision, and fluctuating distance vision." When implanting the rings, the surgeon must not accidentally enter the anterior chamber, which is under pressure. With any operation, the risk of infection is always present.

To a point, increasing amounts of nearsightedness can be treated by using ring segments of greater thickness. A limiting factor in the treatment of larger amounts of myopia is that, once the rings reach a certain thickness, they can interfere with nutrient flow within the eye. Further studies will show how well patients tolerate these inert implants over the long term.

"Orthokeratology," or "Eyebraces"

"Orthokeratology," or ortho-K—the fitting of special contact lenses to alter the curvature of the cornea—does not work well. Results are unpredictable. So save your money. To try to correct nearsightedness, some doctors instruct patients to sleep in specially designed tight contact lenses. Since they have a curvature that is flatter than the cornea, such "eyebraces" push against the gel-like surface epithelium. In the morning, when the patients remove these rigid lenses, their corneas are bent. In other words, they are flatter. But, although ortho-K patients can see better for a few hours early in the day, the effect is only temporary. By about three or four o'clock in the afternoon, the effect has worn off. Part-time "retainer" lenses are required. This is not good medicine! I would never put these contacts on a patient. Since some doctors still fit teenagers with these "orthopedic" lenses, we think people should be told that orthokeratology is not only ineffective, but it is also bad for their eyes.

What is Intra-stromal PRK?

Before LASIK arrived on the scene, doctors dreamed of a perfect "no-touch" laser eye surgery that could remove tissue from the middle, or stromal, layer of the cornea—without disturbing its top layers. Does this sound impossible? It's not. We actually have the advanced laser technology to sculpt the inner cornea without changing the outer layers, but the laws of physics keep "intra-stromal PRK" from becoming a reality. Even though the laser can pass ghost-like through the epithelium and Bowman's membrane, the laser plume, or "exhaust," cannot. As each pulse interacts with stromal tissue, the excimer laser's photoablative byproduct—which looks rather like a tiny, almost invisible, nuclear mushroom cloud—is rapidly ejected. When the laser turns a solid into a gas, the volume increases. Unless this debris can escape into the air, this added volume can produce unpredictable changes in the curvature of the cornea.

So even though we have unprecedented laser optical systems, we lack the answer to a critical question: How can we remove the laser plume from the middle layer of the eye? As one scientist half-jokingly answered: "All we need to do is build a 'smoke stack' in the cornea to let the 'exhaust' pass out of the stroma." Unfortunately, depending on the body's healing response, any such device to expel the laser plume would alter the corneal curvature—and thus its refracting power.

So what is the best way to handle the minute by-products generated with each laser pulse? Create a parallel cut. And that is exactly what LASIK keratomes do. Although the raised flap is not a "smoke-stack," LASIK does allow the laser plume to exit the eye. Scientists have difficult practical problems to overcome before the intriguing concept of intra-stromal PRK—which seems years from becoming a practical reality—can replace LASIK.

EPILOGUE

A human reads letters one by one on the appropriate line on an eye chart from twenty feet. Eagles can see the entire line from at least eighty feet and perhaps much farther.
— "The Sense of Sight," *National Geographic*

Although LASIK won't enable you to see like an eagle, excellent results have significantly improved many people's lives. When patients walk out of our office pleased with their outcomes, we know that we've chosen the right profession. Even after performing tens of thousands of refractive surgeries, I am still thrilled watching the wonder on patients' faces as they look through their laser-treated eyes for the first time. We are absolutely powerless to solve so many problems in ophthalmology, but with LASIK, we have the know-how to help patients see better without corrective lenses. With the new operations, after diagnosing the problem, we can take action to diminish it. The next day, we can see the initial results, and, usually within a few months, the final outcome is apparent.

After LASIK, you and your doctor can grade your results. If a surgeon removes a gallbladder, he can only say, "Well, gee, that was one of the best gallbladders I've ever done." But, after refractive eye surgery, your physician can put you in an examining room and test your eyes. Can you see 20/20, 20/40, or 20/50 the day after LASIK when, before surgery, you were unable to see the big *E?* If you are happy with your results, this is incredibly exciting to both you and your eye doctor.

Though any operation carries some risk, with the latest laser eye surgeries, we have an excellent chance of helping you see more clearly. Many patients achieve 20/20 vision. If only we could help everyone see perfectly. But we cannot make such a pledge. None of us come into this world with a warranty on our body parts or our healing response. As remarkable as modern technology is, it is unable to provide crystal-clear eyesight for every single human being. At present, only a miracle could fulfill such a promise. But then, stranger things have happened.

With time and endless effect, one generation's prayer becomes the next generation's answer.

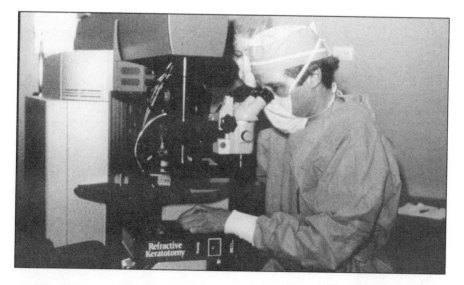

Figure 28

Dr. Slade was the first to perform LASIK in the U.S. with Stephen F. Brint, M.D., under a Summit investigational protocol. (This photograph was taken at another time.)

APPENDIX

The importance of the Munnerlyn formula becomes quickly apparent when you consider how doctors apply it to an individual patient. For example, say someone has a severe -10 diopter refractive error. To create a 5-millimeter optical zone, the surgeon would laser down into the cornea about 100 microns. If the doctor creates a 6-millimeter zone, he will have to laser to 144 microns. For a 7-millimeter zone, to 200 microns. So, the difference between a 5- and a 7-millimeter zone for the same -10 diopter refractive error is twice as deep. Depending on the individual, the center of the cornea is about 550 microns deep, thickening to about 700 microns near the edge. (The horizontal diameter of the cornea is about 12 millimeters and the vertical diameter is 11 millimeters.) Since the higher the myopia, the deeper the ablation, the total depth of the cornea can be the limiting factor that makes some highly myopic patients poor candidates for LASIK. Considering that it is vital to leave an untouched safety net of several hundred microns between the ablation and the corneal endothelium, it is easy to understand why surgeons usually are unable to do laser surgery for people with refractive errors greater than -12 to -14 diopters. For some such patients, the cornea could lack enough remaining supportive tissue.

Some ophthalmologists treat extremely high myopia by using "multizones," whereby more focusing power is put in the inner zone and less in the outer one. In other words, the power of the reshaped lens is stacked in blended concentric circles, or optic zones, that become progressively more shallow toward the edge. Only the central optic zone has 100 percent of the correction. A compromise surgical technique requiring several passes of the laser over the eye, multizone photoablation creates smoothly-blended optic zones of increasing diameters. This operation focuses the patient, limits the depth of the laser ablation, and decreases the amount of tissue removed. The thickness of the lens is reduced. But, although multizones allow doctors to treat higher amounts of myopia, the technique has limits.

GLOSSARY

ablation: vaporization of tissue with the excimer laser during LASIK or PRK.

accommodation: the ability of the human eye to focus close objects (and distant objects for farsightedness). Through the constriction of the ciliary muscles inside the eye and the relaxation of the tiny string-like zonular fibers that are attached to the lens capsule, the elastic crystalline lens inside the eye thickens so that the eye can change focus from distant to near objects. As people age, their accommodative ability decreases, necessitating the need for magnifying glasses or bifocals for close work.

AK (astigmatic keratotomy): a refractive surgical procedure in which a surgeon, using a diamond-tipped knife, makes transverse or arcuate (curved) incisions in the cornea to reduce astigmatism.

ALK (automated lamellar keratoplasty): a refractive surgical procedure to reduce nearsightedness that has been largely replaced by LASIK and PRK. During ALK, a surgeon makes cuts in the cornea with an automated geared microkeratome to decrease the refractive error. Designed after a carpenter's plane, the tiny metal keratome has a sharp blade that makes both the corneal flap and the refractive cut. This non-laser operation can reduce high myopia beyond the range treated with radial keratotomy (RK).

amblyopia: reduced vision typically in one eye with no apparent pathological cause; often called "lazy" eye related to lack of development. Caused by an *imbalance* between the two eyes—either muscular or focusing. Either can lead to the suppression of the vision of the affected eye.

ametropia: a condition denoting a refractive error such as near-sightedness, farsightedness, or astigmatism in which the eye's optical system (without using accommodation) fails to focus the images on the retina for clear vision.

anisometropia: a condition in which there is a significant difference in the refractive power of the two eyes.

anterior chamber: the space near the front of the eye between the cornea and iris filled with a clear circulating fluid called the "aqueous humor."

applanation lens: a special lens used during LASIK allowing the surgeon to measure the proposed diameter of the hinged corneal tissue before it is cut.

aqueous humor: the clear liquid, which is constantly formed and drained from the eye, that circulates through the front chambers of the eye, providing nourishment.

astigmatism [Greek *a* + *stigmata,* "not round"]: a complex refractive error causing blurred vision at every distance, usually because the shape of the cornea is "out-of-round" so that the rays of light fail to come to a focused point on the retina. In regular astigmatism, the more powerful meridian and the least powerful meridian of the cornea are at 90 degrees from one another. The cornea has a smooth optical surface that allows correctable vision with glasses.

atrophy: a loss of function of the eye, or portions of the eye, typically caused by loss of the nerve supply or by an inadequate supply of nutrients.

best-corrected visual acuity (BCVA): the best vision achievable using spectacles or contact lenses.

blepharitis: typically a bacterial infection of the eyelid margins often associated with dry eyes.

Bowman's membrane: the second layer of the cornea that acts as a barrier against infection and trauma. Made of collagen fibrils, Bowman's membrane, which lies between the corneal surface epithelium and the stroma (the middle layer of the cornea), is approximately 12 microns thick. Bowman's does not regenerate.

cataract: a clouding or loss of transparency of the crystalline lens causing mild to severe degradation of vision.

central island: a surgically-induced complication of laser surgery that can occur with the broad-beam excimer lasers. A central island, which can decrease visual acuity, is a raised area on the surface of the central cornea that looks like a small island on a corneal topographical map.

choroid: a vascular structure that nourishes the outer portions of the retina.

ciliary muscle: a muscle inside the eye that controls the focusing power of the crystalline lens. When the ciliary muscle contracts, the tension of the tiny string-like zonular fibers is released, causing the elastic, youthful lens to become thicker (rounder), and thus more powerful to focus close objects.

conjunctiva: the mucous membrane that covers the front of the eyeball and the inside of the eyelids.

conjunctivitis: an inflammation of the conjunctiva mucous membrane that covers the front of the eyeball and the inside of the eyelids. There are many possible causes of conjunctivitis.

contrast sensitivity: a measurement of visual function indicating the ability to discriminate shades of gray.

cornea: the transparent dome-like window of the eye that covers part of the front of the eyeball. The cornea, which consists of five layers—the epithelium, Bowman's membrane, the stroma, Descemet's membrane, and the endothelium, is the eye's most powerful refracting lens. Laser surgery reshapes the cornea to improve vision.

corneal flap: see *flap, corneal*

corneal graft: a transplant operation to rehabilitate vision by replacing layers of a damaged cornea with donor tissue.

corneal topography: the computerized mapping of the surface of the cornea. Color codes represent the various corneal elevations and show the refractive power of the "hills and valleys" of the window of the eye. The changes in the cornea following refractive surgery are apparent on the corneal topographic maps.

corneal ulcer: see *ulcer, corneal*

crystalline lens: the adjustable lens inside the eye that sits about 3 millimeters behind the cornea. This clear flexible lens, which is surrounded by a transparent elastic capsule, has "zoom-lens" capabilities in younger people. Suspended by fine, string-like fibers called "zonular fibers," the crystalline lens can automatically change its shape, becoming rounder to sharpen blurred close images. The shape of this lens is directly controlled by the muscles inside the eye known as the ciliary muscles.

decentration: in refractive laser surgery, a complication that occurs when the excimer laser treatment is off-center. A decentered laser ablation treatment that is improperly placed on the cornea, resulting in a decrease in best-corrected visual acuity (vision with glasses).

Descemet's membrane: the fourth layer of the cornea, lying between the stroma and the endothelium. Formed from secretions from the endothelium, Descemet's membrane, which is 10 to 12 microns thick, serves as the scaffolding for the vital endothelial cells.

diopter: a unit of measurement that delineates the refractive (light-bending, or focusing) power of a lens. The amount of correction needed in glasses or contact lenses to normalize vision is stated in diopters. A lens that can bend parallel light rays to a focal point 1 meter in front of itself is said to have a power of 1 diopter (1D). Twice as strong, a 2-diopter lens can focus light rays at a point 0.5 meters away from the lens. A 0.5-diopter lens is one-half as strong as a 1-diopter lens. Someone with a mildly myopic correction of -1 diopter is focused at 1 meter, or approximately the length of the arm. Someone with a refraction of -2 diopters is focused at 0.5 meters and can see clearly only halfway down the arm. (The reciprocal of the focal distance is a refracting surface.)

emmetropia: normal vision. An eye without refractive errors.

endothelium: the fifth layer of the cornea. A single-cell layer of flat cells that helps control corneal hydration in order to preserve the transparency of the window of the eye. The endothelium, which does not regenerate, serves as a semi-permeable barrier between the aqueous humor in the anterior chamber and the cornea. The metabolic pumping action of the endothelium removes water from the cornea, a process necessary to prevent it from becoming cloudy.

enhancement procedure: a refractive surgical refinement procedure designed to reduce residual focusing errors that sometimes remain after the initial vision correction treatment(s).

epithelium: the first and outer layer of the five layers of the cornea, the clear window of the eye. The gel-like epithelium, which is five to seven cells thick, protects the eye from microorganisms. Epithelial cells normally are replenished about every seven days. If surgically removed, the epithelium grows back in about one to three days.

excimer laser: a cool, invisible ultraviolet laser used to sculpt the human cornea to refocus the eye and thus treat refractive errors such as nearsightedness, farsightedness, and astigmatism. The extremely precise excimer removes tissue at the sub-micron level with virtually no heat or damage to the surrounding tissue.

farsightedness: see *hyperopia*

flap, corneal: the hinged (partially attached) corneal tissue created by the microkeratome during LASIK. The corneal flap protects the lasered middle layer (the stroma) from the air after surgery.

fluence: the amount of energy delivered to a specific area with each pulse of a laser beam. The fluence is the cutting rate of the laser.

fovea: a tiny indention in the macula of the retina that provides the eye's most acute vision. The fovea has a high concentration of light sensitive photoreceptors called cones.

fusion: the brain's ability to receive a slightly different image from each eye and to combine the two images into a single one.

glaucoma: a clinically significant sustained rise in the pressure within the eye that can damage the optic disk and result in a gradual loss of vision and blindness. Some patients have low-pressure glaucoma.

haze: as pertaining to PRK, haze—which often looks like fingerprints on glass when viewed with the slit-lamp microscope—can cloud the cornea, requiring treatment or, when mild, may pass unnoticed by the patient. Haze is seldom a significant problem with LASIK because the protective flap promotes the surgical healing process.

hydrophilic: as pertains to contact lenses, the ability to hold a high water content.

hyperopia (farsightedness): a refractive error in which light passing through the eye's focusing system comes to a theoretical focal point behind the retina if accommodation is completely relaxed. The farsighted eyeball is too short from front to back for the refractive power of the cornea, causing a blurred image of close objects. (The axial length of your eye may be too short, or your cornea may be flatter than normal, or both.)

implantable "contact lenses" (ICLs): also called refractive intra-ocular lenses (IOLs). ICLs are implants, rather than contact lenses. A device to reduce refractive errors such as nearsightedness, an ICL can be surgically implanted inside the eye, either between the iris and the crystalline lens or in the anterior chamber. The natural crystalline lens of the eye remains in place.

intra-ocular lens (IOLs): an artificial lens surgically placed inside the eye. An IOL is used to replace the natural clouded crystalline lens that is removed during cataract surgery.

intra-ocular pressure: the pressure within the globe of the eye caused by the circulating intra-ocular fluids within the front chambers of the eye.

interface: in LASIK, where the repositioned corneal flap meets the surgically exposed inner corneal bed after the excimer laser treatment.

intra-stromal corneal ring segments (ICRS) or Intacs: intra-stromal corneal ring segments are surgically inserted in the cornea to reduce mild amounts of nearsightedness. An ICRS implant, which consists of two transparent, plastic, semi-circular ring segments or arcs, flattens the curvature of the window of the eye. The ring segments can be removed later, if necessary.

iris: a double muscle, the iris is the colored doughnut-shaped diaphragm of the eye that controls the size of the pupil. The iris automatically expands and contracts like a pleated accordion to regulate the amount of light reaching the retina. The color of the iris determines the color of the eye.

irregular astigmatism: astigmatism in which the surface of the cornea is not smooth or the major meridian (the steepest) and minor meridian (the flattest) are not perpendicular to each other. Often caused by a fine wrinkling of the corneal surface, irregular astigmatism, which can be surgically induced, can only be corrected with rigid contact lenses—not with glasses or soft contacts. Surgeons have attempted to diminish irregular astigmatism with some of the newer special lasers with unpredictable results. The advent of the custom "wavefront" LASIK may help some of these patients.

keratectomy: surgically cutting the cornea.

keratitis: an inflammation of the cornea, which may be caused by an infectious agent.

keratoconus: an anomaly or deformity of the cornea in which the cornea becomes cone-shaped and the central area thins. Keratoconus results in irregular myopic astigmatism. Vision can be corrected with specially-ground contact lenses but not with glasses. Progressive keratoconus can eventually cause a loss of the ability to wear a contact lens. In some cases, a corneal transplant may be required to try to restore vision.

keratomileusis: a refractive surgical procedure in which a sliver of tissue of a specified width and thickness, which is flat rather than curved like a lens, is removed from the cornea to correct the refractive error.

The Greek word *keratomileusis* is literally translated as "carving of the cornea." (*Kerato* means "cornea" and *mileusis* means "carving.")

keratotomy: a surgical procedure (such as radial keratotomy) in which incisions are cut in the cornea.

lamellar surgery: an operation performed within and between the thin collagen layers (lamellae) of the cornea.

LASIK (*laser in situ keratomileusis or laser assisted in situ keratomileusis*): a microsurgical refractive procedure, LASIK, which is outpatient laser surgery, reduces or eliminates refractive errors such as nearsightedness, farsightedness, or astigmatism. During LASIK, a specially trained surgeon, working under a thin corneal tissue flap, uses a computer-controlled excimer laser to reshape the human cornea, changing its curvature. After a preprogrammed amount of lens-shaped tissue is removed from the middle layer of cornea, the doctor lays the protective hinged flap back over the laser-treated area.

microkeratome: a small metal surgical instrument used during LASIK and some other refractive procedures to gain access to the middle layer (the stroma) of the cornea. Functioning rather like a carpenter's plane, a microkeratome, or keratome, which has an exquisitely sharp blade, is an extremely precise device that cuts a preset amount of tissue from the cornea to create a hinged flap.

micron: a unit of measurement. One micron equals one-millionth of a meter.

minification effect: a visual effect whereby objects appear smaller than they are.

miotic agent: an ophthalmic drug that constricts the pupil.

monovision: a way of managing age-related presbyopia, whereby one eye is focused for distance and the other eye is at least partially focused to improve near vision. A goal of monovision is to improve near vision with or without bifocals.

mydriatic agent: a pupil-dilating drug that makes the pupil larger.

myopia: nearsightedness. It is a refractive error in which parallel light rays come to a focus in front of the retina, instead of directly on it. A nearsighted person can see better close up than in the distance.

nearsightedness: see *myopia*

nomogram: an algorithm, or mathematically derived table, of refractive surgical parameters consulted by the surgeon to achieve a specific correction.

ophthalmologist (oculist): a medical doctor (M.D.) who specializes in the diagnosis and treatment of diseases, conditions, and refractive errors of the eye. An ophthalmologist writes prescriptions and performs surgery.

optic disk: insensitive to light, the optic disk, which is sometimes called the "blind spot," is the head of the optic nerve where the retinal nerve fibers come together. As seen with the ophthalmoscope, the optic disk normally looks like a pink depression or cup.

optic nerve: the nerve that transmits visual impulses to the brain from the retina.

optician: a specialist who fits, makes, and dispenses glasses and contact lens.

optometrist: a licensed eye-care professional trained to examine the eye for defects and other conditions. Optometrists measure refractive errors and write glasses prescriptions. Optometrists (O.D.'s) are doctors of optometry. They do not perform surgery.

overcorrection: in refractive surgery, an overcorrection occurs when the cornea receives too much treatment so that images are not focused directly on the retina of the eye. When a nearsighted eye is surgically overcorrected (or heals in an unexpected way), the person can become farsighted if the cornea becomes so flat that images fall behind the retina instead of on it.

pachymeter: an instrument used to determine the depth of parts of the eye. Key to refractive surgery, an ultrasound pachymeter can measure the thickness of the cornea.

phacoemulsification: a surgical technique used to remove a cataract (a clouded crystalline lens). An ultrasonic needle breaks up the cataract, and the fragments are aspirated through a little hole in the instrument. A foldable replacement lens implant, or intra-ocular lens (IOL), replaces the clouded lens. A stitch to close the incision usually is unnecessary.

phakic: an eye that has its natural crystalline lens. (An aphakic eye has no crystalline lens.)

photoablation: in refractive eye surgery, the extremely precise vaporization or removal of layers of corneal tissue with the excimer laser to improve vision.

photoreceptors: consisting of the rods and the cones, the photoreceptors of the retina make up part of the light-gathering neural circuitry of the brain.

posterior chamber: the fluid-filled hollow space behind the colored iris and in front of the crystalline lens. The posterior chamber of the eye contains circulating aqueous fluid, which is under pressure.

PRK (photo-refractive keratectomy): a microsurgical surface procedure that uses an excimer laser to correct refractive errors such as nearsightedness and astigmatism. After removing the thin gel-like outer coating (the epithelium) from the window of the eye, the surgeon reshapes the cornea with the computer-controlled excimer laser. Results are dependent on the wound-healing response and on the regrowth of the epithelium.

phoropter lens: an instrument with rotating dial-up lenses used to measure refractive errors and other problems in order to write a prescription for glasses or contact lenses.

plano: without any refractive light-bending power or dioptric power; a flat (not curved) piece of glass or plastic with no light-focusing capability.

presbyopia: literally, "old eyes." Presbyopia, which usually starts to become noticeable around age forty, occurs because the crystalline lens behind the pupil gradually loses its ability to focus close objects (to accommodate). People with presbyopia usually wear magnifying glasses or bifocals to read.

pupil: the dark center of the eye. The size of the light-gathering pupil is controlled by the surrounding iris rather like the aperture of a camera is determined by the size of its diaphragm. The pupil expands in dim light to let more light reach the retina and contracts in bright light to protect the retina from excessive stimulation.

radial keratotomy (RK): an incisional refractive surgical procedure to reduce or eliminate nearsightedness by flattening the curvature of the dome-shaped cornea, or window of the eye. Using a guarded diamond-tipped knife, a specially trained surgeon makes fine spoke-like incisions in the cornea to change its focusing power by weakening the peripheral cornea.

refraction: in ophthalmology, measuring the focusing error of the eye to prescribe glasses or contact lenses to correct nearsightedness, farsightedness, astigmatism, or age-related presbyopia.

refractive error: a flaw in the eye's ability to focus light directly on the retina for clear vision. The major refractive errors are nearsightedness, farsightedness, astigmatism, and age-related presbyopia.

refractive surgery: in ophthalmology, any operation, such as LASIK, PRK, or RK, performed to reduce or eliminate refractive errors including nearsightedness, farsightedness, astigmatism, or age-related presbyopia (with monovision).

regression: after refractive surgery, any change in refractive power that reverses the initial outcome of the procedure. After PRK, for example, initially-corrected nearsightedness may partially return, negating some of the surgically-induced improvement in visual acuity.

residual hyperopia: the amount of farsightedness remaining after refractive surgery.

residual myopia: the amount of nearsightedness remaining after refractive surgery.

retina: containing the light-receiving photoreceptors (the rods and the cones) of the brain, the retina is the inner coating of the back of the inside of eyeball. Like the film in a camera, the retina is exquisitely sensitive to light. Unlike film, the retina, which is necessary for sight, cannot be replaced.

retinal detachment: a serious condition in which the retina separates from the back of the eye causing symptoms such as a dark "curtain" falling over all or a portion of the visual field.

Schirmer's test: a test that measures the volume of tears in the eyes. Doctors use the Schirmer's test to diagnose dry eyes.

slit-lamp microscope: a powerful microscope with a special light source used to view the structures of the eye under magnification.

Snellen eye chart: consisting of letters, numbers, and even symbols, the Snellen eye chart (it has the big *E* at the top) is used to measure central visual acuity (VA). By ascertaining the smallest figures that one can distinguish at a specified distance, an eye doctor can assess VA. Patients who can read the 20/20 line at 20 feet have normal visual acuity. Those who read the 20/40 line at 20 feet see at 20 feet what normally sighted persons see at 40 feet. VA as measured by the Snellen eye chart cannot be *accurately* converted to diopters.

sclera: the opaque white part of the eye.

spherical aberration: a distortion of images that occurs with high-power lenses. Light rays coming through either side of such a highly curved lens are bent progressively more than those coming through the center. The latter are parallel. For example, glasses for severe nearsightedness fail to focus bundles of light coming in through the edges at the same point as light coming through the center. Although modern lens-grinding techniques decrease spherical aberration, glasses with large amounts of correction still can distort vision.

stereopsis: three-dimensional depth perception, or binocular vision, occurs because each eye sees an object from a slightly different angle.

strabismus: caused by a muscle imbalance, strabismus occurs when the two eyes fail to look directly at an object at the same time resulting in loss of binocular vision. The wayward eye is sometimes called the "lazy," or crossed, eye.

stroma: the third, or middle, layer of the cornea, forming about 90 percent of its thickness. Consisting of "lamellar" layers made of collagen fibers, the transparent stroma is about 80 percent water. The stromal lamellae, which are stacked in clear horizontal tiers rather like the layers of an onion, are specifically arranged in a geometrical design that allows the uninterrupted passage of the visible wavelengths of light.

stroma remodeling: the body's restructuring of the third layer of the cornea (the stroma) after refractive surgery that can cause regression of the effect of the procedure, especially following PRK.

subconjunctival hemorrhage: a blood-filled swelling located beneath the conjunctiva, the membrane that lines the inside of the eyelids and the front part of the eye, except the cornea.

tear film: a three-layer fluid film that moistens the cornea and the conjunctiva. Vital to the health of the cornea, the tears supply dissolved oxygen from the air to the window of the eye.

tonometer: an ophthalmic instrument used to measure the pressure within the eye.

20/20 vision: normal vision, or visual acuity as measured by the Snellen eye chart that accesses the smallest object a person can see clearly at a distance of 20 feet. Someone with 20/20 visual acuity can read the 20/20 line on the eye chart at 20 feet. Someone with 20/40 sitting 20 feet from the chart is only capable of seeing the larger figures on this line that the person with normal vision sees 40 feet away. Although eye charts vary, usually someone with 20/400 visual acuity sitting 20 feet away from the eye chart can only read the giant *E* at the top.

ulcer, corneal: a serious infection of the cornea that can lead to progressive tissue destruction (necrosis). An ulcer, which can have many different causes, must be treated immediately.

undercorrection: in refractive surgery, a result after treatment in which the eye is not corrected enough to attain normal distance vision. An undercorrection may be planned or unplanned.

visual acuity: as measured by the Snellen eye chart, a person's clearness of vision, or ability to discern letters and figures at a specified distance. Normal, or emmetropic, visual acuity is called 20/20 vision.

visual axis: the line-of-sight connecting the retinal fovea (the area of most acute vision) with the object of regard.

vitreous: the transparent, viscous fluid that fills the chamber of the eye behind the crystalline lens. Surrounded by the retina, the thick jelly-like vitreous, which contains the shock absorber called hyaluronic acid, is almost 99 percent water.

zonular fibers: the tiny, string-like, suspensory ligaments, whose tension is controlled by the ciliary muscles, determine the thickness and thus the refractive power of the crystalline lens. To see close objects, the zonular ligaments relax, and the flexible lens assumes its natural round shape.

RESOURCES

American Academy of Ophthalmology

P.O. Box 7424

655 Beach Street

San Francisco, CA 94120

Ph: 415-561-8500

Website: www.eyenet.org

American Optometric Association

1505 Prince Street, #300

Alexandria, VA 22314

Ph: 703-739-9200

Website: www.aoanet.org

American Society of Cataract and Refractive Surgery

4000 Legato Road, Suite 850

Fairfax, VA 22033

Ph: 703-591-2220

Website: www.ascrs.org

International Society of Refractive Surgery
1175 Spring Center South Boulevard, #152
Altamonte Springs, FL 32714
Ph: 888-813-4777
Website: www.isrs.org

TECHNICAL MEDICAL BOOKS ON EXCIMER LASER SURGERY AND RK

The Art of LASIK
Jeffery J. Machat, M.D., and Stephen G. Slade, M.D.
SLACK Inc., 1998
Thorofare, NJ

Atlas of Refractive Surgery
Benjamin F. Boyd, M.D.
SLACK Inc., 1999
Thorofare, NJ

LASIK
Ioannis Pallikaris, M.D., and Dimitrios Siganos, M.D.
SLACK Inc., 1997
Thorofare, NJ

LASIK Complications: Prevention and Management
Howard V. Gimbel, M.D.
SLACK Inc., 1999
Thorofare, NJ

LASIK: Principles and Techniques
Lucio Buratto, M.D., and Stephen F. Brint, M.D.
SLACK Inc., 1998
Thorofare, NJ

Refractive Keratotomy for Myopia and Astigmatism
George O. Waring III
Mosby-Year Book Inc., 1992
St. Louis, MO

Refractive Surgery
Helen K. Wu, Vance M. Thompson, Roger F. Steinert,
Stephen G. Slade, and Peter S. Hersh
Theime, 1999
New York & Stuttgart

Refractive Surgery
Dimitri T. Azar, M.D.
Appleton & Lange, 1997
Stamford, CT

Equipment Manufacturers

Aesculap-Meditec
23832 Via Monte
Coto De Caza, CA 92679
Ph: 714-589-6259

Autonomous Technologies Corp.
520 North Semoran Boulevard, Suite 180
Orlando, FL 32807
Ph: 407-282-1261

Bausch & Lomb Surgical (Chiron Vision Products)
555 West Arrow Highway
Claremont, CA 91711
Ph: 909-624-2020

Coherent Medical
3270 West Bayshore Road
P.O. Box 10122
Palo Alto, CA 94303-4043
Ph: 650-858-2250

EyeSys Vision Group/Premier Laser Systems Inc.
3 Morgan
Irvine, CA 92618
Ph: 800-544-8044

LaserSight Technologies Inc.
12249 Science Drive, Suite 160
Orlando, FL 32826
Ph: 407-382-2700

Nidek Inc.
47651 Westinghouse Drive
Fremont, CA 94539
Ph: 510-226-5700

Novatec Laser Systems Inc.
2237 Faraday Avenue
Carlsbad, CA 92008
Ph: 760-438-6682

Summit Technology
21 Hickory Drive
Waltham, MASS 02154
Ph: 781-890-1234

Sunrise Technologies
47265 Fremont Boulevard
Fremont, CA 94538
Ph: 510-623-9001

VISX Inc.
3400 Central Expressway, Suite 101
Santa Clara, CA 95051
Ph: 408-733-2020

NATIONAL LASER CENTERS

The Laser Center Inc. (TLC)
A publicly-traded company, TLC, headquartered in Mississauga, Ontario, represents six thousand doctors who share information, monitor quality control, proctor results, and review difficult cases. There are TLC centers throughout the U.S. Dr. Jeffery J. Machat and Dr. Stephen G. Slade are the national medical co-directors of TLC.

U.S. toll-free number: 1-888-CALLTLC
Canadian toll-free number: 1-800-TLC-1033
Website: www.lzr.com

ClearVision Laser Centers Inc.

ClearVision Laser Centers Inc., headquartered in Lakewood, Colorado, has affiliated surgeons in more than eighty-five communities in Colorado, Idaho, Indiana, Georgia, Michigan, Nevada, Pennsylvania, Tennessee, Utah, and Washington.

Toll-free number: 1-888-464-2020
Website: www.clearvisionlaser.com

Laser Vision Centers

Laser Vision Centers, headquartered in St. Louis, Missouri, provides access to lasers, focusing on small- and medium-sized markets.

Toll-free number: 1-888-LASERVISION
Website: www.laservision.com

VIDEOS

The Role of Optometry in Refractive Surgery
Richard N. Baker
Patient Education Concepts, 1995.

Eyelearn LASIK
Stephen G. Slade, M.D.
Digital Interactive Computerized Education Inc., 1996.
Santa Monica, CA

CD-ROMs

Eyelearn LASIK
Stephen G. Slade, M.D.
Digital Interactive Computerized Education Inc., 1996.
Santa Monica, CA

BIBLIOGRAPHY

Books

Buratto, Lucio, and Stephen Brint. *LASIK: Principles and Techniques.* Thorofare, N.J.: SLACK Inc., 1998.

Casebeer, Charles J. *Casebeer Incisional Keratotomy.* Thorofare, N.J.: SLACK Incorporated, 1995.

Casebeer, Charles J., L. Ruiz, L., and Stephen G. Slade. *Lamellar Refractive Surgery.* Thorofare, N.J.: SLACK Inc., 1996.

Hubel, David H. *Eye, Brain, and Vision.* New York: Scientific American Library, 1988.

Machat, Jeffrey J. *Excimer Laser Refractive Surgery.* Thorofare, N.J.: SLACK Inc., 1996.

Machat, Jeffrey J., and Stephen G. Slade. *The Art of LASIK.* Thorofare, N.J.: SLACK Inc., 1998.

Nordan, L., A. Maxwell, and J. Davison, eds. *The Surgical Rehabilitation of Vision.* New York: Gower Medical Publishing, 1992.

Poole, Robert M., ed. *The Incredible Machine.* Washington, D.C.: National Geographic Society, 1986.

Rozakis, G., S. Hollis, F. Kremer, and Stephen G. Slade. *Refractive Lamellar Keratoplasty.* Thorofare, N.J.: SLACK Inc., 1994.

Stein, Slatt, and Raymond M. Stein. *The Ophthalmic Assistant. 6th ed.* St.Louis: Mosby-Year Book Inc., 1994.

Thornton, Spencer P. *Radial and Astigmatic Keratotomy.* Thorofare, N.J.: SLACK Inc., 1994.

Waring, George O. III. *Refractive Keratotomy for Myopia and Astigmatism.* St. Louis: Mosby-Year Book Inc., 1992.

Zajonc, Arthur. *Catching the Light.* New York: Oxford University Press, 1993.

CHAPTERS IN BOOKS

Ruiz, L., Stephen G. Slade, and Stephen Brint. "Excimer Laser Keratomileusis" in *Corneal Laser Surgery.* St. Louis: Mosby-Year Book Inc., 1995.

Slade, Stephen G. "Lamellar Refractive Surgery" in *Refractive Surgery.* Appleton Lange, 1994.

Slade, Stephen G., L. Ruiz, and S. Updegraff. "Corneal Topography in Lamellar Refractive Surgery" in *Corneal Topography: The State of the Art.* Thorofare, N.J.: SLACK Inc., 1995.

COURSES

Casebeer, Charles J., and Stephen G. Slade. *LASIK Course Manual.* Chiron Vision Corp., 1995.

Casebeer, Charles J., and Stephen G. Slade. *Lamellar Refractive Surgery Course Manual.* Chiron Vision Corp., 1996.

VIDEOS

Baker, Richard N. *The Role of Optometry in Refractive Surgery.* Patient Education Concepts, 1995.

Slade, Stephen G. *Eyelearn LASIK.* Santa Monica: Digital Interactive Computerized Education, Inc., 1996.

CD-ROMs

Slade, Stephen G. *Eyelearn LASIK.* Santa Monica: Digital Interactive Computerized Education Inc., 1996.

SELECTED JOURNAL ARTICLES

Baker, Richard N. "How to Screen Candidates for Refractive Surgery." *Review of Optometry.* (1995).

Brint, Stephen J., and Stephen G. Slade. "Six Month Results of the Multicenter Phase I Study of Excimer Laser Myopic Keratomileusis." *Journal of Cataract and Refractive Surgery.* 20 (1994): 610–615.

Donaldson, S. L., G.H. Strauss, and Stephen G. Slade. "Use of Tissue Adhesive (Tiseel) in Epikeratophakia." *Investigative Ophthalmology and Visual Sciences.* 31, 4 (1990): 30.

Martone, J., S. Holland, Stephen G. Slade, S. Laukaitis, and O. Foot. "Project Orbis." *International Ophthalmolgy Clinics.* 30, 1 (1990): 58.

Ruiz, L., and Stephen G. Slade. "Form Meets Function." *Eyecare Technology.* 5, 2 (1995): 67–69.

Slade, Stephen G. "The Case for Corneal Transplantation in Developing Countries." *Refractive and Corneal Surgeries.* 7, 6 (1991): 477–78.

Slade, Stephen G. "Interview: Automated Lamellar Keratoplasty." *Ocular Surgery News.* 11, 8 (1993): 69.

Slade, Stephen G. "Treatment for High Myopia." *In Visionary.* Summit Technology Visionary Program (1994).

Slade, Stephen G. "Lamellar Refractive Surgery." *Seminars in Ophthalmology.* 9, 2 (1994): 117.

Slade, Stephen G. "Automated Lamellar Keratoplasty." *Ocular Surgery News.* 12 (1994): 14.

Slade, Stephen G. "Phase I Excimer ALK Results." *Ocular Surgery News* 12 (1994): 19.

Slade, Stephen G. "Automated Lamellar Keratoplasty with the Summit Excimer Laser." *European Journal of Implant and Refractive Surgery.* 6 (1994): 232–236.

Slade, Stephen G. "Sur Le Fil Du Rasior." *Abstract Optalmo.* 1, 1 (1995): 15–18.

Slade, Stephen G. "Two Views on Laser In-Situ Keratomileusis." *ARGUS.* 19, 1 (1996): 20–21.

Slade, Stephen G., J.F. Gordon, P.A. Lee, and R.M. Dru. "A Prospective Multicenter Clinical Trial to Evaluate Lamellar Keratoplasty for Myopia." *Investigative Ophthalmology and Visual Science.* 35, 4 (1994): 2156.

Slade, Stephen G., and S.A. Updegraff. "Advances in Lamellar Refractive Surgery. International Ophthalmolgy Clinics." 34, 4 (1994): 147, 163.

INDEX

ABOUT THE AUTHORS

Stephen G. Slade, M.D., FACS

A world's leading expert in refractive surgery, Stephen G. Slade, M.D., FACS, helped develop LASIK—the state-of-the-art laser vision correction eye surgery that is practiced worldwide today. He was the first to perform this procedure in the U.S. with Stephen F. Brint, M.D. Dr. Slade has surgically corrected tens of thousands of nearsighted, farsighted, and astigmatic patients and has trained virtually all of the surgeons performing LASIK in the U.S. today.

A master cataract and corneal surgeon, Dr. Slade has served on the faculty of the Department of Ophthalmology at the University of Texas Medical School and on the Food and Drug Administration (FDA) investigatory eye care technology panel that evaluates the introduction of new technologies in the U.S. He is the chair of the Refractive Surgery Section of the American Society of Cataract and Refractive Surgery. He has served as the treasurer of the International Society for Refractive Surgery and the medical director for Project Orbis, the flying eye hospital.

Dr. Slade has received numerous honors, including the 1986 Outstanding Young Houstonian Award, the 1996 Refractive

Surgeon of the Year Award, the 1997 LANS Lectureship, and the Honor Award of the American Academy of Ophthalmology. The People's Republic of China honored him for his service in fighting blindness by twice presenting him with the China Service Medal.

An international lecturer and prolific writer, Dr. Slade has co-authored five medical books on refractive surgery, including *The Art of LASIK*, the leading medical text in the field. He also has written many scientific articles and book chapters.

He is the lead investigator for many innovative technologies, such as microkeratomes to create the surgical flap for LASIK and a new implantable, flexible cataract replacement lens to correct age-related presbyopia. This operation has the potential to reduce dependence on reading glasses for millions of older people. The ophthalmologist has invented specialized surgical instruments and has three U.S. patents pending for refractive surgery.

Dr. Slade is the Medical Monitor for the Bausch & Lomb Technolas Excimer Laser and is the National Medical Director for The Laser Center (TLC), a company representing six thousand doctors who share information, monitor quality control, proctor results, and review difficult cases.

A Phi Beta Kappa graduate of the University of Texas, Dr. Slade received his M.D. from the University of Texas Medical School in Houston, Texas, where he was president of his class. He was chief resident at Louisiana State Eye Center in New Orleans, Louisiana, and was a corneal fellow for Project Orbis in New York. He also was a corneal fellow at Baylor College of Medicine, Houston, Texas.

Richard N. Baker, O.D., FAAO

Richard N. Baker, the Director of The Laser Center of Houston, is a faculty member for Bausch & Lomb Chiron Ophthalmics, the LASIK Advanced Course. He has spent almost his entire professional career caring for tens of thousands of refractive surgery patients.

Dr. Baker has presented lectures on LASIK to eye doctors all over the world.

A 1975 graduate of the University of Houston College of Optometry, Dr. Baker has been a co-investigator for the Summit Laser. He has helped Dr. Slade direct LASIK training courses for ophthalmologists in the U.S.

Dorothy Kay Brockman

Dorothy Kay Brockman, a freelance writer who lives in Houston, Texas, was a patient of Dr. Slade who experienced the miracle of LASIK surgery. She is the author of several books on medicine and computers, including *In Pursuit of Fertility*, which she co-authored with Robert R. Franklin, M.D., clinical professor, Baylor College of Medicine. As a LASIK patient, she understands the emotions and stresses of undergoing refractive eye surgery.